Yogaflows™

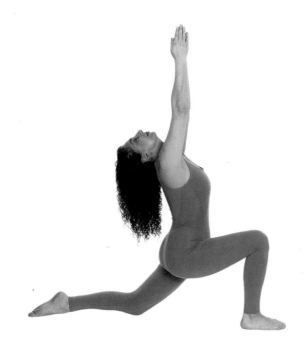

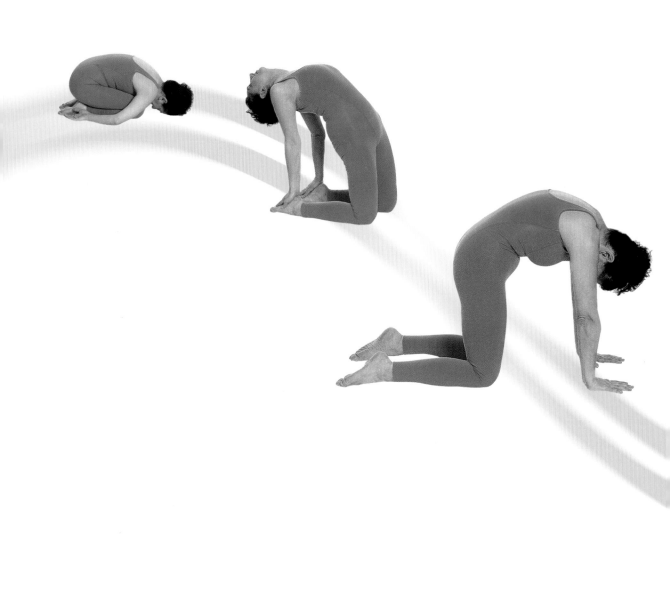

Yogaflows™

A dynamic and fluid system
to transform your yoga practice

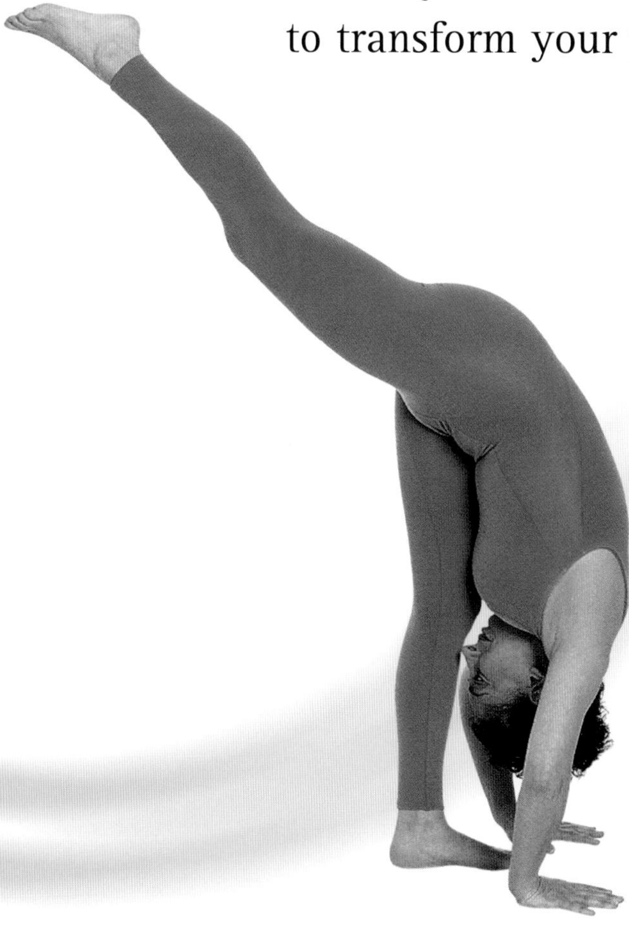

MOHINI CHATLANI

FIREFLY BOOKS

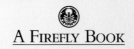

A FIREFLY BOOK

Published by Firefly Books Ltd., 2003

Created and produced by
Carroll & Brown Publishers
20 Lonsdale Road Queen's Park
London NW6 6RD

First Printing

National Library of Canada Cataloguing in Publication Data
Chatlani, Mohini
Yogaflows: A dynamic and fluid system to transform your everyday
yoga practice/Mohini Chatlani.
Includes index.
ISBN 1-55297-687-4
1. Yoga, Hatha. I. Title.

RA781.7.C43 2002   613.7'046   C2002-902716-0

U.S. Cataloging in Publication Data (Library of Congress Standards)
Chatlani, Mohini.
Yogaflows: A dynamic and fluid system to transform your yoga practice/Mohini Chatlani—1st ed.
Originally published: U. K.: Carroll & Brown, 2002.
[144] p.: 550 col. photos; 24.6x18.9 cm. Includes index.
Summary: Hatha yoga presented in a series of sequential poses for all levels of yoga practitioner.
ISBN 1-55297-687-4 (pbk.)
1. Yoga, Hatha. I. Title.

613.7/ 046 dc 21   RA781.7.C53   2003

First published in Canada in 2003   First published in the United States in 2003
by Firefly Books Ltd.   by Firefly Books (U.S.) Inc.
3680 Victoria Park Avenue   P.O. Box 1338, Ellicott Station
Toronto, Ontario M2H 3K1   Buffalo, New York 14205

Editor Anna Amari-Parker
Art Editor Evie Loizides-Graham
Photographer Jules Selmes

Reproduced by Colourscan, Singapore
Printed in China for Imago

Disclaimer: This book is not a medical, therapeutic, or remedial resource. If you are ill, injured
or have a medical condition, please seek professional medical advice before beginning any of the
practices outlined herein. The author and publishers disclaim any liability from any injury
occurring in the practice of the programs outlined in the book.

contents

foreword

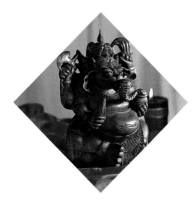

Affectionately known as Ganpathi, the elephant god Ganesh is the bestower of boons, the remover of obstacles and the herald of new beginnings. Powerful yet compassionate, his large belly indicates his ability to "stomach" anything.

Yoga is much more than just an excellent physical exercise. It is an ancient and powerful spiritual tradition aimed at transforming an inaccurate perception of reality into a clear perception of that which is real. It is able to elicit in you a global loving-kindness which will help you become a better participant in life.

The title of the book says it all: yoga flows. And yoga flows because life flows. Life is the flowing movement of ever-new creation and yoga is the realization of this unalterable fact and this unstoppable energy.

Learning to flow through the practice of yoga helps you attune to the harmonious flow of life itself. The more congruent you are with the inexhaustible flow of creation and of life, the more harmony, health, peace of mind and fulfillment you will experience and exude.

This is the whole point of yoga: what is good for the self becomes beneficial to those who surround you. Learning to flow through the practice of yoga is most assuredly life-affirming and positively invigorating.

I have been friends with Mohini for several years now and I know she has put her whole heart into writing Yogaflows *and it shows. There is a lot of expressed joy here. You can see it in Mohini's face and read it in Mohini's words.*

In Yogaflows, *you will find a wealth of information and years of intuitive practice distilled into suggested practice routines. The 12 flow sequences included in this book are fun, intelligent and effective. Learn them, tune into the source of their creation and become the place where joy flows through.*

With love and pranams,

Erich Schiffmann

an inspired practice

Yogaflows is a fully illustrated, easy-to-follow guide created and compiled to introduce a unique and fluid system of practicing classical yoga. It offers a dynamic approach to *hatha* yoga.

As it may at first be difficult to establish your own personal practice when you are learning classical *hatha* yoga, each of the 12 yogaflows in this book contains different, creatively sequenced yoga poses originating and distilled from ongoing experiential and spontaneous personal practice. The flows move from one pose to the next, linked by conscious, rhythmic *Ujjayi* (victory) breath to create *vinyasas* (dynamic breathing flows). With practice, dedication and a sense of humor, these sequences may be learned so that the poses become part of a creative series rather than remaining isolated, individual poses.

Finding a middle ground

The key to yogaflows is threefold: breath, body and awareness. Focusing on your breath becomes the fulcrum from which to observe your body. The breath effectively ignites all *asanas* (poses), bringing them to life. Being present at every moment invites you to internalize attention; nurture self-reliance; take responsibility for your thoughts, words and deeds; acquire patience and tolerance toward yourself and others; increase self-acceptance; develop an awareness of criticism, competitiveness, judgments and attachments; note comparisons between yourself and others. Through this inner awareness, you are able to embrace yourself with greater compassion and, in so doing, encourage meeting others in the same way.

Although there is external movement in yoga practice, yogaflows promotes calmness within in the form of dynamic meditation. It helps you find a subtle balance

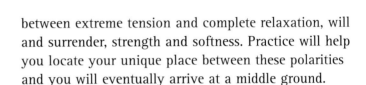

between extreme tension and complete relaxation, will and surrender, strength and softness. Practice will help you locate your unique place between these polarities and you will eventually arrive at a middle ground.

External and internal form

This may shift from day-to-day and from moment-to-moment throughout your life as you continue to change internally. You may need to be willful and strong in your practice initially, concentrating largely on external form (technique, alignment, precision and conscious effort). This will engage your body and mind until they become familiar with the various poses and the sequences. As your practice develops, your body will become stronger, resulting in a stabilization of the poses and a more focused mind.

Your awareness of internal changes will be enhanced. This will enable you to recognize that it is energy which moves your body, rather than muscular strength. Attention and presence need to be maintained at every breath, heightening your senses so that your body learns to move with effortless ease. You begin to observe your experience while holding each yoga pose, almost as if you were a witness, without the need to be judgmental.

In the flowing structure of yogaflows, there is an absence of struggle or competition as you move from one pose into another. Poses become more than just a collection of actions, and a balance is maintained between the inhalation and the exhalation.

The fusion of mind, breath, energy and movement results in a vibrant and energetic union of inner and outer environments. From here, you can tap into and experience deeper states of awareness or consciousness.

The synergy of breath, body and observation moves you into an awareness of the subtler movements of energy or the *prana* (life force). Here you are able to access your inner world through the external, creative expression of yogaflows.

Mind and body

By working with the *prana,* you begin to regenerate energy around your body. As the subtler energy is harnessed, a still, focal point of attention may be felt within.

Both mind and body can directly experience physical sensations as they are received—undiluted, away from conditioned mindsets, fears and resistance. The body is able to dance or flow with grace, beauty and elegance. The mind merges with an all-encompassing awareness in an experience of transcendence which is energetic and ecstatic.

Yogaflows encourages a release of the conditioned mind, enhancing a continuous moment-by-moment awareness which brings you back to the "here and now". With practice, your mind learns to relax.

Criticism, judgments, attachments and anxieties begin to diminish as the movements of your body ride on the wave of awareness, fueled by the breath which is energy in motion. Strength may be powered by energy, but there is also the art of effortless flexibility. Even as your body comes to external stillness for meditation, there is continuous movement occurring within. This is the paradox of yoga: externally still, yet internally dynamic; externally dynamic, yet internally still.

Letting yoga into your life

Ancient and traditional yoga practices can easily be adapted to the rhythms of modern-day life and serve as effective tools in changing the way you think and feel. You come to the practice of yoga with your own emotional and mental baggage. The more burdens you carry and the constant retelling of your personal story reinforces your sense of feeling alienated, and adds unnecessary emotional weight to your life. The result is a feeling of separation from, rather than one of being connected with all living things.

Greater self-awareness

When using yoga as a self-generated system of healing, your body effectively becomes like a barometer. As you tune into yourself, you will learn to read the signs that reflect your emotional, mental and spiritual states. This internal state is then reflected back to you through the mirror of your external environment and you begin to see a very different picture of yourself. You move closer to merging with your true self to realize your inner strength. As the *prana* (life force) pervading you and the entire planet awakens, the *shakti* (innate spiritual power) also begins to stir.

Yoga is a means of opening up to your body and your heart with compassion. It not only develops strength, flexibility and sensitivity, but also provides you with a means for deepening your awareness, innate knowledge and energy. It helps build up core strengths and values, encourages self-reliance, perseverance, compassion, self-empowerment and unconditional love.

As form is de-emphasized through the practice of yogaflows, you come deeper into the *asanas* (poses) and learn to tune into intuitive movement, showing you the potential for a new relationship with yourself. As a result, you learn to move from within to without. This teaches you the dynamics of harmonizing with those around you. You learn to take responsibility for yourself in the poses and thus in your life.

Learning to let go

By respecting your body and trusting it a little deeper each time, you learn humility in accepting your limitations. Through physical and energetic intimacy with yourself, you prepare to move into intimacy with another. Observe the daily build-up of tensions, blocked by conditioned mindsets. As you move through these physical blocks, you encounter their mental counterparts. This allows you to discard the mask you wear and moves you into a freer expression of who you are, with greater self-awareness, confidence and joy. Learn to transform the negative feelings of conflict, isolation, loneliness, fear, guilt, blame, co-dependency and shame which alienate you from your True Self and impede your full realization as an individual.

Yogaflows promotes the ultimate union of breath, movement and awareness. The synergy of these elements can essentially only occur through experiential practice rather than intellectual study, making yoga a very individual and intensely transforming experience.

yoga with a difference

Traditionally, yoga *asanas* (poses) were taught and practiced individually. In some disciplines, *asanas* were alternated with periods of *Savasana* (Corpse) to experience a calming effect on the mind: the "stress response" was reversed in favor of the "relaxation response".

The nature of yogaflows is inherently dynamic. This is a noticeable departure from standard *asana* practice where a continuous dynamic flow enhances vascular circulation either by moving from one *asana* into another with only one breath per pose, or by holding each pose for several breaths before moving on to the following pose. Linking them in a flowing sequence emphasizes the continuous, steady rhythm of movement and breath. The practice, although dynamic and flowing, is sometimes challenging, although never strenuous or vigorous. It integrates periods of rest, observation, breathing practices and a variety of yoga-related techniques, which encourage you to practice at your own pace so you can tailor your practice to suit your prevailing energy levels and physical state at a given time.

Classical *hatha* yoga does not employ *Ujjayi* (victory) breath during active *asana* practice. Traditionally, it is used as a *pranayama* (breath control).

Yogaflows uses *Ujjayi* breath as an integral part of the practice, encouraging *pratyahara* (internalization of the senses), *ekgrata* (focused attention) and *dharana* (concentration). As a result, experience and practice are enhanced.

how to use this book

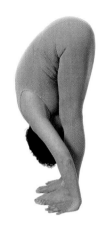

Yogaflows is structured in three sections which correspond to three different levels of yoga expertise—basic (levels one and two), moderate and intensive. Each section is preceded by a selection of carefully selected warm-up exercises. Practice these before doing any yogaflows. Each warm-up section is accompanied by instructions which guide you smoothly from one level to the next. If you have an existing knowledge of breathing techniques and yoga poses in general, but are not familiar with the original idea of yogaflows, you may wish to start at the simplest level. Once you have grasped the general idea, simply select any of the yogaflows. Always practice on empty bowels and bladder, use a yoga mat and, if tired, take it easy. Wear loose, comfortable, cotton clothes.

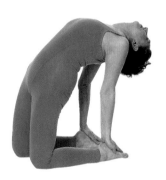

There is a natural progression through the book regarding levels of yoga practice: sequences become increasingly complex. First, look at the images to familiarize yourself with the dynamism of a given flow. Then, read the instructions relating the two. If any of the poses are particularly challenging or new to you, refer to the Glossary (*see page 120*), where a detailed description of all 123 poses featured may be found. Within some of the yogaflows you will also find a diamond icon referring you to the Focus on Flows section (*see page 100*), where additional instructions and images will closely guide you through the more difficult poses.

The inspirational quotes accompanying each yogaflow have arisen intuitively and spontaneously either from my own personal practice or during my yoga classes. They may be used simply to inspire general practice, as a means of accessing deeper individual responses, or as themes for meditation and relaxation.

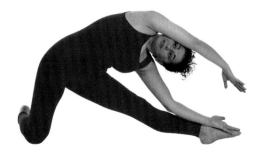

benefits of yogaflows

Each yogaflow sequence harnesses the benefits of each of the poses it contains by coupling breathing technique with general awareness. This modifies the energy which moves through different areas of your body, helping to clear tensions and energy blocks.

Once the movement of energy is activated through physical exercise in the yogaflow sequences, an internal gate is opened to release this spontaneous, energetic flow. One of the benefits of free-flowing internal energy is to detoxify and heal the body's systems.

Although each yogaflow can be practiced separately, they work together as a complete healing unit to leave you feeling relaxed and revitalized with a sense of inner calm. Your senses are heightened: hearing, sight, sense of touch all become more acute (as does your understanding) and a greater sense of well-being is felt.

The practice of yogaflows promotes a moment-by-moment awareness that enables you to remain grounded in the "here and now". This concentration is greatly encouraged and will, through practice, eventually filter into your daily life. When successfully applied, it will enable you to remain focused on the task at hand.

Through heightened awareness of the inhalation and the exhalation, breathing becomes circular and seamless, which encourages a fully relaxed functioning of your lungs and promotes general well-being. Taking in the breath is saying "yes to life", to being infused with the *prana* (life force), which enables you to transmute inert, habitual ways of being into dynamic, energized and focused living.

yoga is an internal journey
to the magic
of becoming
light and empowered

preparing for yogaflows practice

Before starting your practice, sit quietly in a comfortable, seated position for a few minutes to center and ground your body and connect with your natural, flowing breath. Remain in the present moment by coming back to an awareness of your breath.

Once your natural breath is regular and you are aware of it, begin to deepen your breath by focusing it at the nostrils. As rhythm is established, introduce *Ujjayi* (victory) breath (*see pages 42–43*). Use this practice throughout each yogaflow, gradually establishing a feel for middle breathing (*see pages 86–87*).

During your practice, become aware of your pelvic floor through the practice of *bandhas* or energy body locks (*see pages 64–65*). Softly draw the muscles of your perineum inwards and upwards, to engage *Moola Bandha* (Root or Perineum Lock). An awareness of firming up your lower abdomen from hip to hip is also recommended through modified *Uddiyana Bandha* (Lower Abdominal Lock).

Start each of the yogaflows on your right side, resting in *Savasana* (Corpse) or *Gharbhasana* (Child) between sides, if necessary. Then repeat each flow on your left side.

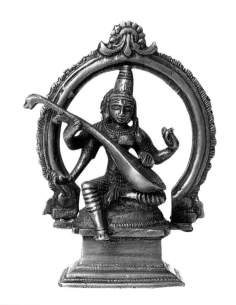

Originally known as the River Goddess, Saraswati means 'the watery one'. Initially the goddess of speech and learning, the representation of Saraswati eventually came to encompass all creative art forms—poetry, art and music. She is well known for bestowing her grace on all those who invoke her.

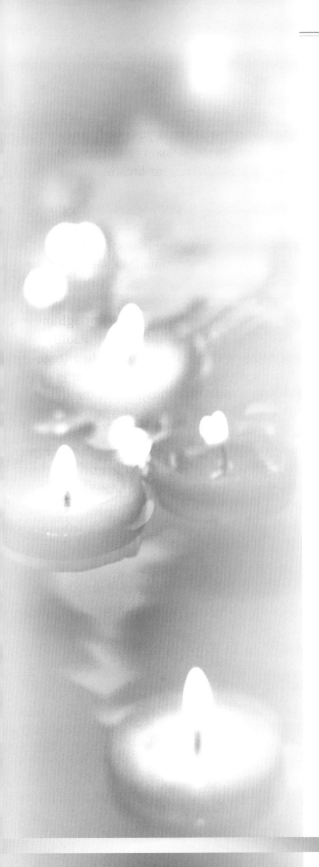

Respect and listen to your body, never pushing it into discomfort. Move gently into your stretch, becoming accustomed to feeling your "edge"—the spot where, if you went further, pain would occur. Learn to hold your stretch, sometimes softening, sometimes deepening it. Increase your "edge" without strain. Hold the poses only for as long as is comfortable. The guidelines in yogaflows suggest one breath in, one breath out while holding a pose. However, poses can be held for any number of comfortable breaths. It is a self-elective method.

Be guided by your inner movement and the mood of a given moment. Once familiar with yogaflows, choose a piece of music to suit your frame of mind. Music stimulates the right-brain hemisphere and helps clear your mind, allowing you to relax and ease yourself into your practice. Experiment and see the difference. The choice is yours!

guidelines for warm-ups

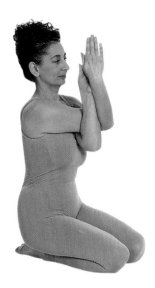

Warm-ups, as the name implies, increase body temperature, producing heat, energy and relieving soreness and tightness in aching joints or muscles. They increase your pulse rate, raise your body's core temperature, oil your joints, and oxygenate and elasticize muscles and tissues. The Fire breath used in dynamic warm-ups is designed to energize, bringing instant heat to muscles and joints and increasing energy flow. Warm-ups build up strength, endurance, determination, self-reliance and prepare your body for *asana* practice.

Where there is dynamic movement, coordinate the motion of your body, or body parts, with your breath as indicated. Repeat each warm-up several times before moving on to the next one, staying present and focused on your experience. Unless otherwise specified, use *Ujjayi* breath throughout. When doing a series of warm-ups on one side or leg, remember to rest between sides, observing the differences that occur when switching from side to side.

Following recent surgery or illness, consult your physician before starting practice. If you are pregnant, remember never to use Fire breath during your pregnancy. Avoid compressing your abdomen and do not forget to widen the gap between your legs when doing Standing Forward Bends and *Gharbhasana* (Child). As your pregnancy progresses, many poses will not be possible, so relaxation, breathing, visualization and meditation practices will be of the utmost benefit.

Inverted poses and Fire breath are not recommended for women who are menstruating, or for anyone with high blood pressure or a heart condition. Use soft *Ujjayi* breath and practice slowly. Do not rush the movements and even slow them down if necessary.

helping yourself through yoga

If you have recently had surgery, have a condition or weakness in any part of the body, or are pregnant, consult our chart to familiarize yourself with the types of *movement currently most beneficial to you through yoga practice. Outlined below are these different types of movement and their respective benefits.*

Types of movement	Practice carefully with a weakness in the body parts below	Avoid with any of the injuries or conditions below	Benefits
Backward-bending Spine-arching	Use *Moola Bandha* (Root or Perineum Lock). Hold poses for shorter periods. Arch your back less.	Spine: invertebrated hernia (slipped disk); heart and blood conditions; high blood pressure; ankylosing spondylitis; spondylarthritis; lumbar spondylosis; abdominal conditions.	Strengthens the spine. Energizes and revitalizes the body. Builds self-confidence and courage. Helps to dispel fear and anxiety.
Forward-bending Spine-folding	Bend your knees with lower back pain.	Acute sciatica; invertebrated hernia (slipped disk); acute spinal conditions.	Massages the abdominal organs. Stimulates circulation. Calms the mind and the emotions.
Head-lowering Inversions	Medicated high blood pressure; low blood pressure. Avoid holding poses for long periods. Lift your head.	Heart, blood or circulatory conditions; stroke patients; high blood pressure; thrombosis; epilepsy; menstruation; vertigo; hiatus hernia; detached retina; glaucoma; ear and eye conditions.	Detoxifies the body. Enhances the endocrine system. Improves thinking and concentration.
Twist Lateral side-bending Abdominal-compressing	Compress lightly.	Pregnancy; menstruation; hiatus hernia; diverticulitis; gastritis; severe back and abdominal conditions.	Twist and abdominal: Aids digestion and stimulates the spine. Detoxifies and decongests. Lateral: Improves breathing and spine and hip alignment.
Knee-bending Standing Balance	Bend your knees less.	Knees: osteo–rheumatoid arthritis; bursitis.	Improves coordination, balance and endurance. Energizes and calms the nervous system.
Knee-compressing Knee-pressing	Use padding under your knees.		
Wrist-flexing	Use your fists or forearms. Avoid holding poses for long periods.	Wrists, elbows, arms, hands and fingers: osteo–rheumatoid arthritis; Carpal Tunnel syndrome.	Improves wrist articulation and mobility.
Neck-arching Neck-compressing	Do not overarch your back. Lengthen your neck. Keep your head straight.	Hyperthyroidism; cervical or lumbar spondylosis; ankylosing spondylitis.	Improves spinal alignment and circulation to the brain. Stimulates the neck and throat.

getting ready to flow
basic warm-ups

Warm-ups (see pages 18–19) serve as gentle body stretches which can de done in isolation from one another and are often dynamic in nature. Begin each warm-up below slowly. Gradually develop your awareness and deepen your breath where necessary, eventually picking up the pace. Hara warm-ups (see pages 44–47) will specifically warm and energize your body. The rest of the warm-ups are generally useful for stretching muscles and loosening up stiffened joints.

1 STICK

Lie with your body flat on the ground, legs together, feet flexed, arms by your sides, palms down. Reach your arms up beyond your head, pressing the small of your back into the ground as your whole body stretches out, feet pointing away. Exhaling, bring your arms back down by your sides, feet flexed, palms down. Repeat dynamically several times.

2 SIT-UP I

Lie with your body flat on the ground, arms along the sides, legs apart. Exhaling, bring your right knee to your chest as your torso comes up to meet your knee. Lift up your arms and left leg, keeping them parallel to the ground, feet flexed. Hold. Release and repeat with your left leg.

3 BRIDGE

Lie in a semi-supine position with your knees bent, feet flat, away from your buttocks, arms down by your sides. Inhaling, press into your feet as you lift your hips, buttocks, pubis and abdomen and raise your arms up above your head, tucking your tailbone in. Exhaling, bring your arms back and your body down. Repeat dynamically several times.

4 CAT AND DOG TILT WITH VARIATIONS

Come down on all fours, knees hip-width apart, wrists beneath your shoulders, knees beneath your hips, back flat. Press your hands into the ground and round your back as your tailbone drops down (*pose a*). Hold. Return to starting position.

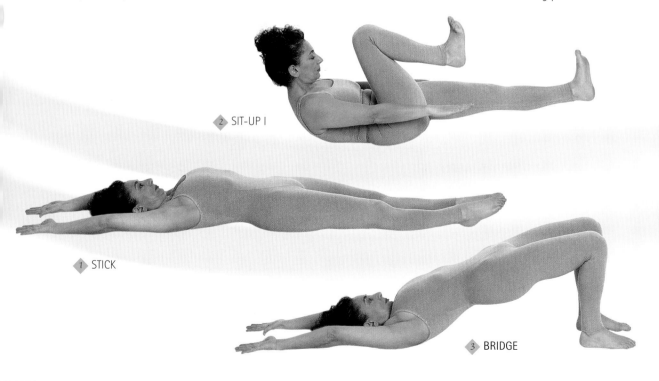

2 SIT-UP I

1 STICK

3 BRIDGE

Press your hands into the ground and let your tailbone rise as your back arches and your head lifts (*pose b*). Hold. Return to starting position. Move dynamically between Dog and Cat Tilt.

Return to starting position and prepare to move your body, starting from your hips. Circle your hips around dynamically in one direction a few times, then the other.

Return to starting position. Turn your head and look over your right shoulder, keeping your ear close to your shoulder. Draw your right hip toward your head, stretching out your left side. Use "ha" breath. Repeat on your left side.

5 HEAD-TO-KNEE WITH VARIATIONS

Come down on all fours, knees hip-width apart, wrists beneath your shoulders, knees beneath your hips, back flat. Lift your right leg up behind your body as you arch your back. Lift up your head. Round your back as you bring your head to your right knee. Go back and forth dynamically in both directions. Use "ha" breath. Repeat with your left leg.

Come down on all fours. Lift up your right leg behind your body. Keeping your right leg up, begin pulsing it up and down. The action should come from your hip. Use a soft, panting breath "ha, ha, ha" with a soft, natural inhale. Repeat with your left leg.

Come down on all fours. Lift up your right leg behind your body. Hold it up and engage your right hip in a circling motion, initially rotating with small, then gradually larger, circles. Repeat with your left leg.

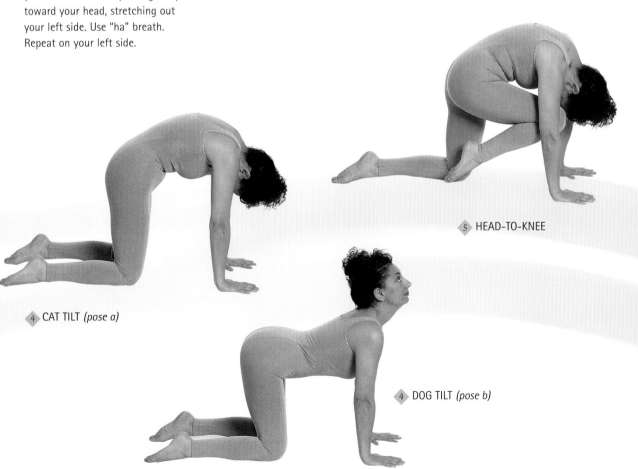

4 CAT TILT *(pose a)*

5 HEAD-TO-KNEE

4 DOG TILT *(pose b)*

6 ½ THREADING-THE-NEEDLE
Come down on all fours, knees
hip-width apart, wrists beneath
your shoulders, knees beneath
your hips, back flat. Exhaling,
thread your right arm through the
gap between your left knee and
left hand. Bring the back of your
head and shoulder down to the
ground. Return to starting position.
Thread your left arm through. Repeat
dynamically, holding it on one side,
then the other.

7 EAGLE
Sit back on your heels, knees
together. Cross your right arm over
your left, lifting your forearms up in
front of your face. Bring your palms
as close together as you can. Hold.
Lift your arms up as high as you
can. Hold. Move your arms around in
a circular motion, as your body
follows the movement. Repeat,
reversing arms, with your left arm
over your right.

8 PRAYER
Sit back on your heels, knees
together. Bring your arms up
behind your back, palms together.
Allow your little fingers to move
slowly up your back. Open your heart
as you draw your shoulders back. If
your palms do not reach, hold your
elbows behind your back until your
shoulders loosen up.

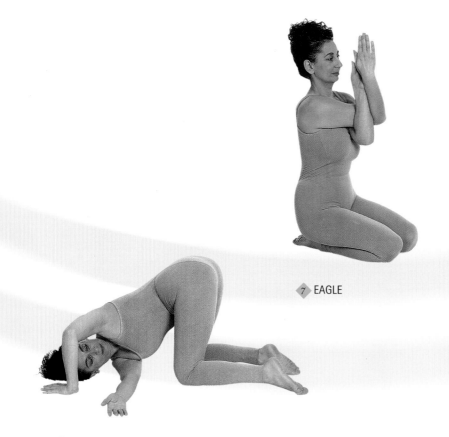

7 EAGLE

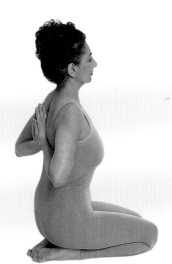

6 ½ THREADING-THE-NEEDLE

8 PRAYER

9 FORWARD FOLD I

Sit back on your heels, knees together. Bring your arms up behind your back, palms together. Exhaling, lower your torso down to your thighs. Bring your head to the ground. Return to starting position. Repeat, reversing arms if you have been holding your elbows.

10 SHOULDERS

Sit back on your heels, knees together. Take your left arm behind your back as your right arm reaches up, elbow bent. Take your right hand down behind your back and grasp your left wrist, hand or fingers. If your hands do not reach, use a yoga strap, tie, or a sock between each hand until your shoulders relax. Repeat, reversing arms.

11 FORWARD FOLD II

Sit back on your heels, knees together. Take your left arm behind your back as your right arm reaches up, elbow bent. Take your right hand down behind your back and grasp your left wrist, hand or fingers. Exhaling, fold your upper body over your thighs and bring your head down to the ground. Exhaling, come up and release. Repeat, reversing arms.

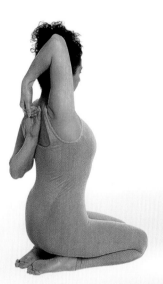

10 SHOULDERS

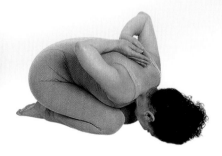

9 FORWARD FOLD I

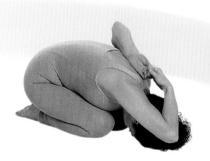

11 FORWARD FOLD II

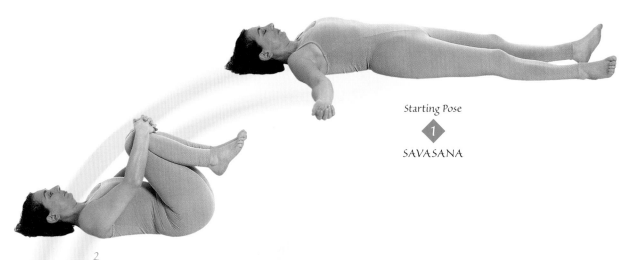

Starting Pose

1

SAVASANA

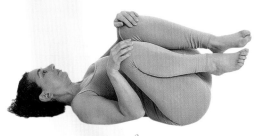

2

JANU
JHULANASANA

yoga is an invitation to wholeness
an invocation to our inner glory
a call for it to emerge
a beckoning for us to see
the invitation is yours

3

JANU
MANDALASANA

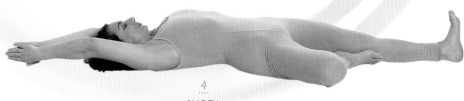

4

SUPTA
VRKSHASANA

1 Inhale. Exhaling, lie in *SAVASANA* (Corpse). Use *Ujjayi* breath.

2 Inhale. Exhaling, bring your knees to your chest. Interlock your fingers around the outside of your knees. Begin gently rocking from side-to-side in *JANU JHULANASANA* (Sacral-Rocking).

3 Inhaling, place your hands on top of your knees. Circle your knees in one direction, then the other, in *JANU MANDALASANA* (Knee-Circling).

4 Inhale. Exhaling, bring your feet down and extend your left leg, foot flexed. Inhaling, place the sole of your right foot along your left inner thigh, lifting your arms over your head, hands in Namaskara (Salutation), in *SUPTA VRKSHASANA* (Supine Tree).

5 Inhale. Interlock your fingers, turning your palms away. Exhaling, hold your right knee and bring it to your chest. Inhale. Repeat, lifting your arms overhead. Release your right leg, feet pointed. Exhaling, return your arms and right knee to your chest, feet flexed in *PAVANMUKTASANA I* (Wind-Relieving I). Repeat for 3–5 rounds.

6 Inhale. Repeat (5). Then exhaling, bring your head to your knee in *PAVANMUKTASANA II* (Wind-Relieving II).

7 Inhale. Exhaling, bring your arms to shoulder level on the ground. Lie on your left side. Align shoulder, hip, knee and ankle. Inhale, place your right foot on your left knee. Exhaling, bring your right knee down to the left. Keep your right shoulder grounded. Place your left hand on the outside of your right knee. Extend your right arm out at shoulder level. Turn your head to the right in *SUPTA MATSYENDRASANA* (Supine Knee-Down Twist).

8 Inhale. Exhaling, return to Savasana (Corpse). Exhaling, bend your left leg and place your foot on the ground. Exhaling, bend your right knee. Take hold of your right foot with both hands, fingers interlocked around the sole of your foot. Keep your sacrum grounded. Exhaling, bring your knee down to the outside of your chest toward the ground. Keeping your elbows bent with your right elbow on the outside of your right leg, bring your foot up, parallel to the sky, calf and thigh at right angles in *SUPTA EKAPADASANA* (Supine Single-Leg Reclining Lunge).

9 Exhaling, release your foot. Place it on your left thigh, sole facing up. Hold your right foot with your left hand. Rest your right hand on your right knee. Inhaling, bring your knee toward your chest. Exhaling, press your knee down, opening your groin and hip in *SUPTA ARDHA PADMASANA* (Supine Half-Lotus).

10 Inhale. Exhaling, release your foot, placing your left hand on your left thigh. Hook your right big toe with the index and second finger of your right hand. Inhale. Exhaling, extend your leg upward and straighten it in *SUPTA PADANGUSTHASANA* (Supine Hand-to-Foot).

11 Inhale. Exhaling, release your toe, keeping your leg extended and your foot flexed upward. Place your arms, palms down, on the ground at shoulder level. Begin circling your leg around the axis of your hip in *SUPTA UTTANPADASANA/MANDALASANA* (Supine Single-Leg Raising/Circling). Repeat in both directions on the same leg. Release.

12 Inhale. Exhaling, bring the soles of your feet down to the ground, slightly away from your buttocks. Exhaling, press your feet down as your pelvis and pubis rise. Moving up, raise your arms beyond your head. Inhale. Exhaling, bring your arms back and your pelvis down. Tuck in your tailbone, your abdomen in Cat Tilt, aligning each of your vertebrae. Coordinate your arms and pelvis on the exhale in *SETHU BANDHASANA* (Bridge).

13 Inhale. Exhaling, lower your body to the ground and bring your legs up to perpendicular. Lift your torso toward your legs, arms parallel. Release on the exhale in *MANIPURASANA* (Abdominal). Repeat the whole yogaflow sequence on your other side.

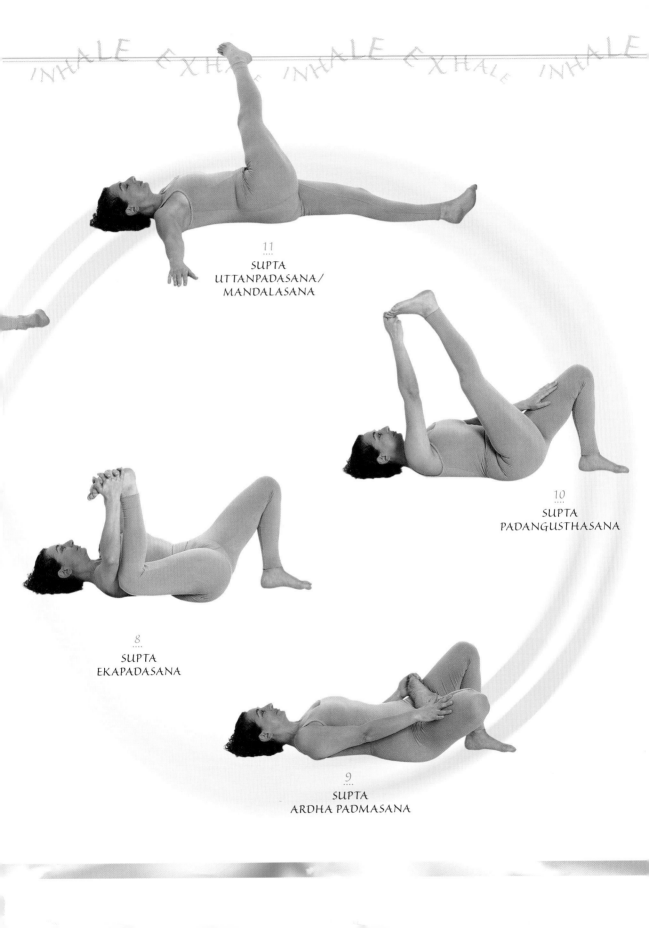

11
SUPTA
UTTANPADASANA/
MANDALASANA

10
SUPTA
PADANGUSTHASANA

8
SUPTA
EKAPADASANA

9
SUPTA
ARDHA PADMASANA

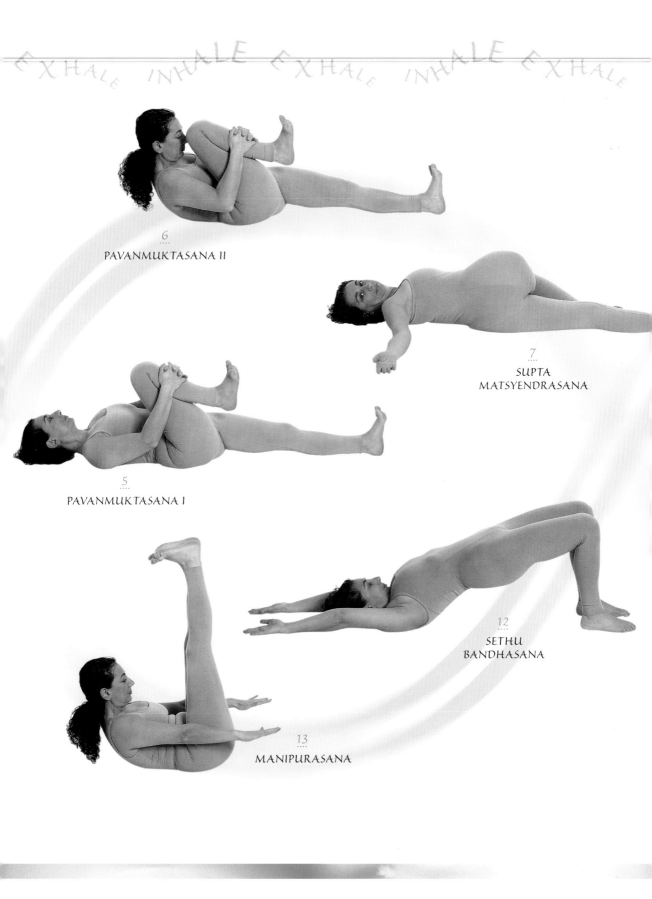

EXHALE INHALE EXHALE INHALE EXHALE

6
PAVANMUKTASANA II

7
SUPTA
MATSYENDRASANA

5
PAVANMUKTASANA I

12
SETHU
BANDHASANA

13
MANIPURASANA

yogaflow
basic level one 2

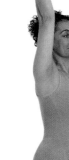

2
....
TALASANA I

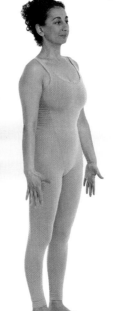

Starting Pose

TADASANA I

3
....
TALASANA II

4
....
TALASANA III

1 Inhale. Exhaling, stand in TADASANA I (Mountain I) with your feet hip-width apart.

2 Inhaling, come up on tiptoes as your right arm lifts up vertically in front of your body. Exhaling, rotate your arms backward as your heels meet the ground in TALASANA I (Mountain I Variation). Coordinate the return of your arms and your heels with your breath. Repeat with your left arm.

3 Inhaling, repeat (2) with both arms in TALASANA II (Mountain II Variation).

4 Inhaling, come up on tiptoes. Lift both your arms up horizontally, bringing palms together above your head. Exhaling, rotate your arms backward as your heels return to the ground in TALASANA III (Mountain III Variation).

5 Inhaling, cross your arms in front of your pelvis, raising your crossed arms up vertically in front of your body, above your head, coming up on tiptoes for a fuller stretch. Exhaling, rotate your arms backward and return them to the front of your pelvis, arms crossed in the opposite direction in TALASANA IV (Mountain IV Variation). Repeat.

6 Inhaling, lift your arms up to horizontal, at shoulder level, in front of your body. Exhaling, bend your knees to descend to a squatting position as if to sit

down on a chair. Keep your torso upright in UTKATASANA I (Standing Squat I). Inhaling, release your knees and come back up. Exhaling, bring your arms down by the sides of your body.

7 Inhaling, lift your arms up to horizontal, at shoulder level, in front of your body. Come up on tiptoes and look ahead. Exhaling, still on tiptoes, bend your knees down to a squat in UTKATASANA II (Standing Squat II). Inhaling, release your knees and come back up. Exhaling, bring your arms down by the sides of your body.

8 Inhale. Exhaling, lift both arms vertically, above your head, as you raise your right leg in front of your body in UTHITTA EKAPADASANA I (Raised One-Foot I).

9 Inhale. Exhaling, move your right leg backward as your arms come to horizontal, palms down, right foot flexed. Tip your body forward horizontally as far as you can, keeping both hips aligned, in UTHITTA EKAPADASANA II (Raised One-Foot II). Inhale. Exhaling, return to Tadasana I (Mountain I).

10 Inhale. Exhaling, lift your arms out to the sides, above your head. Interlock your palms and press them upward in TADASANA III (Mountain III).

11 Inhale. Exhaling, bring your arms down as your right knee comes up to your chest. Hold your knee, your palm faces the inside of your knee in STHITHI PAVANMUKTASANA I (Standing Wind-Relieving I).

12 Inhale. Exhaling, bring your left hand to your left hip, still holding your right knee with your right hand. Inhale. Exhaling, rotate your right knee out to the side in STHITHI PAVANMUKTASANA II (Standing Wind-Relieving II).

13 Inhale. Exhaling, return your right knee to the center. Place your right foot along your left inner thigh as high up as you can. If you are new to this pose, remember that the lowest point your right foot can be is with your right big toe firmly placed on the ground, your foot flat along your heel and ankle, your right knee pointing outward. As your balance progressively stabilizes, your foot can be moved gradually up your leg and into the inner thigh of your left leg. Inhaling, bring your hands into Namaskara (Salutation) and either hold your hands in front of your heart (a), on top of your head (b), or in full pose, stretched out beyond your head (c) in VRKSHASANA (Tree). Inhale. Exhaling, bring your arms down, releasing your foot. Stand in Tadasana I (Mountain I). Repeat the whole yogaflow sequence on your other side.

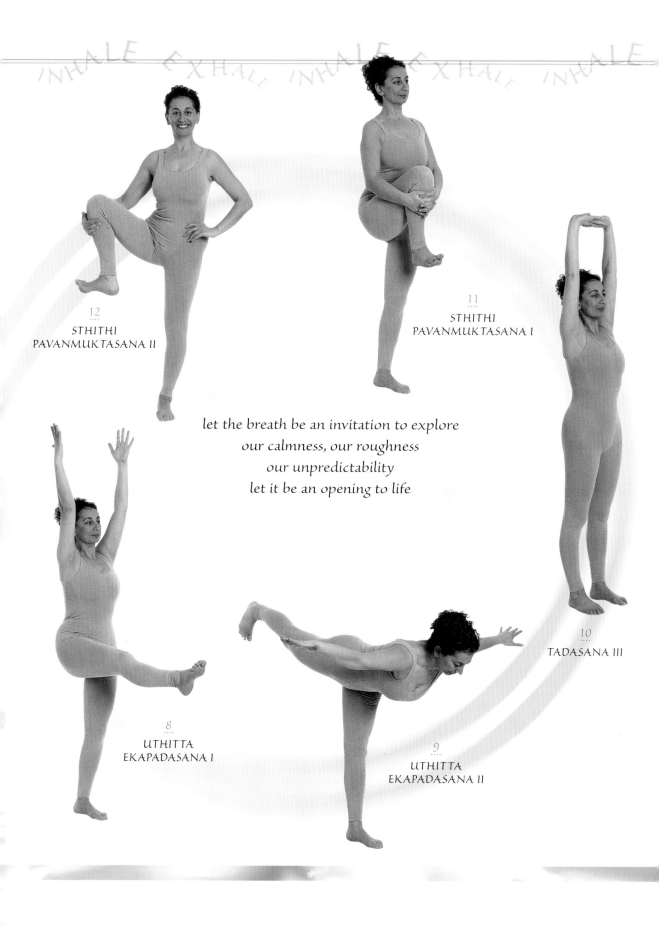

12
STHITHI
PAVANMUKTASANA II

11
STHITHI
PAVANMUKTASANA I

let the breath be an invitation to explore
our calmness, our roughness
our unpredictability
let it be an opening to life

10
TADASANA III

8
UTHITTA
EKAPADASANA I

9
UTHITTA
EKAPADASANA II

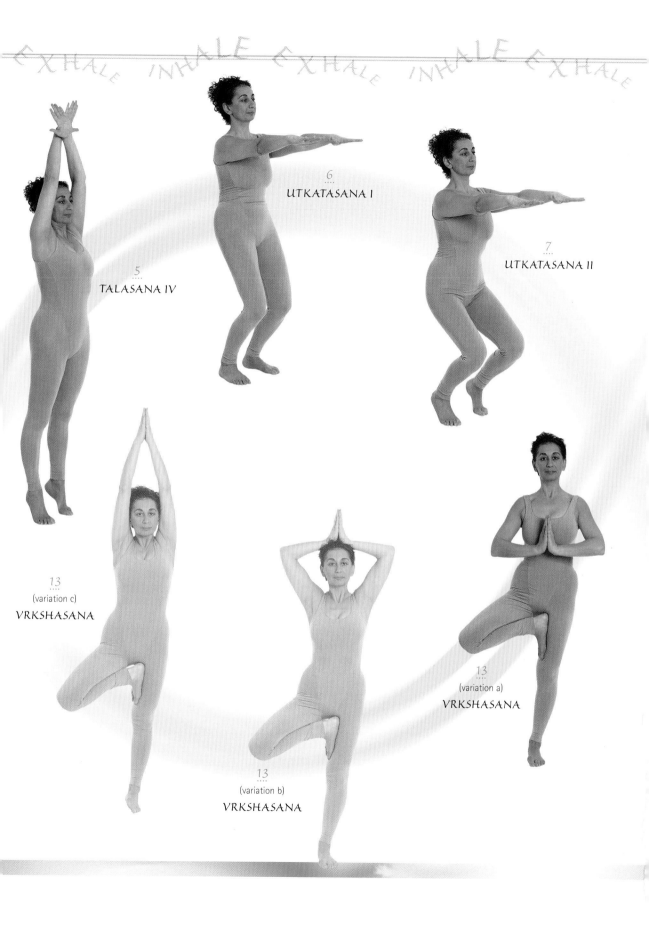

6
UTKATASANA I

7
UTKATASANA II

5
TALASANA IV

13
(variation c)
VRKSHASANA

13
(variation a)
VRKSHASANA

13
(variation b)
VRKSHASANA

yogaflow
basic level two 3

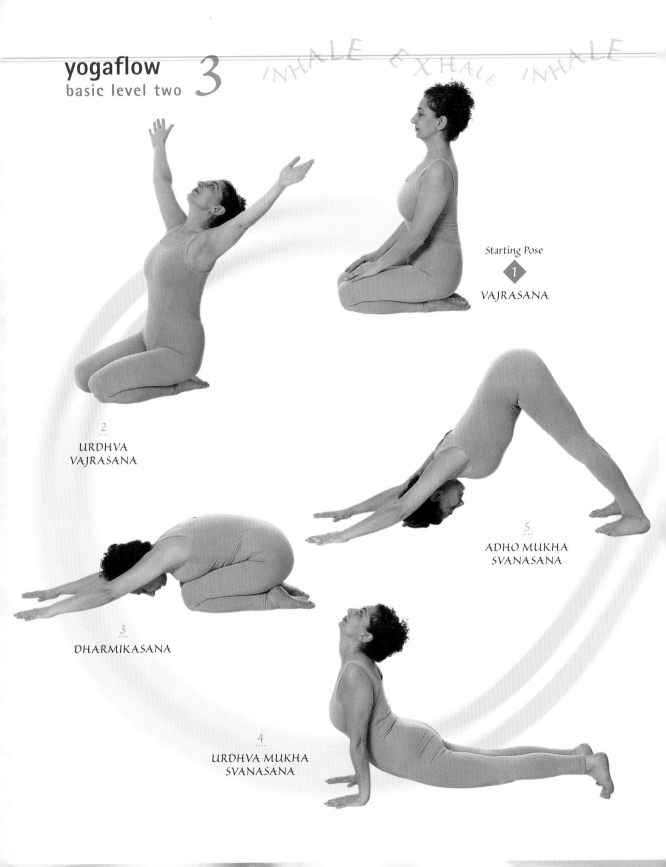

Starting Pose
1
VAJRASANA

2
URDHVA
VAJRASANA

3
DHARMIKASANA

4
URDHVA MUKHA
SVANASANA

5
ADHO MUKHA
SVANASANA

1 Inhale. Exhaling, stand in TADASANA I (Mountain I).

2 Inhaling, raise your arms alongside your ears in TADASANA II (Mountain II).

3 Inhale. Exhaling, bring your feet a little closer together. Interlock all fingers except your index fingers which extend up and cross your thumbs. Inhale. Exhaling, press your left hip out as your body leans over to the right in ARDHA CHANDRASANA I (Half-Moon I).

4 Exhaling, return to Tadasana II (Mountain II). Inhaling, bend your left knee, taking your body weight onto your left foot. Draw in your right foot in front of your left. Exhaling, lift your right leg off the ground, your inner thigh and calf facing upward, right foot flexed. Inhale. Exhaling, bring the back of your right hand to your forehead. Rest the back of your left hand in front of your navel, elbows bent in NATARAJASANA II (Dancer II).

5 Inhaling, open your arms and right leg outward. Exhaling, bring your right foot down, bend your knees down to a squat, arms bent at the elbows in DEVIJAI UTKATASANA (Victory Goddess Squat).

6 Exhaling, straighten your arms and legs. Turn your hands inward and backward, palms face backward in PANCHANGASANA (Five-Pointed Star). Your body

"looks" like a cross or a star with opposite arms and legs creating a diagonal and a cross at the heart.

7 Inhaling, turn your left foot in, right foot out. Keep your arms out horizontally, at shoulder level, legs straight. Exhaling, reach over to the right. Keeping your spine straight, tilt your arms downward. Your right palm reaches toward your leg, foot or ground on the inside of your right foot. Extend your left arm up vertically in UTHITTA TRIKONASANA (Extended Triangle). Look up.

8 Inhaling, come up. Exhaling, turn your head to the right. Look along your right arm as you bend your right leg to a right angle in VIRABHADRASANA II (Warrior II).

9 Inhale. Exhaling, turn your head to the center as your right leg straightens. Bring your hands to your hips, feet parallel. Inhale, look up. Exhaling, fold your body forward and place your palms or fingertips in the space between your feet in line with their arches. If possible, bring the top of your head to the floor in PRASARITA PADOTTANASANA (Spread-Leg Forward Fold).

10 Inhaling, turn both your feet and torso to the right. Exhaling, tuck your back toes into the ground. Bend your right knee to a right angle, placing both palms on the ground, either side of your right

foot. Extend your back leg and knee. Inhale. Exhaling, press your hips and pelvis down to the ground as you stretch your groin area in ASHWA SANCHALASANA II (Rider's II High Lunge).

11 Inhale. Exhaling, lift your tailbone as you step your right foot back, feet parallel in ADHO MUKHA SVANASANA (Downward-Facing Dog).

12 Inhale. Take your body weight forward, supporting it on your hands and toes. Exhaling, lower your pelvis in URDHVA MUKHA SVANASANA (Upward-Facing Dog).

13 Inhale. Exhaling, release your knees down to the ground. Relax your feet, drawing your buttocks toward your heels. Bring your hands by your ankles, releasing your arms, shoulders and forehead to the ground in GHARBHASANA (Child).

14 Inhale. Lift your head. Exhaling, bring your hands down in front of your knees. Tuck in your toes. Exhaling, press into your hands and toes to raise your knees. Lift your body upward, walking your hands back into PADA HASTASANA (Standing Hand-to-Foot Forward Fold). Inhaling, start to uncurl your body, allowing your head to come up last. Exhale. Repeat the whole yogaflow sequence on your other side.

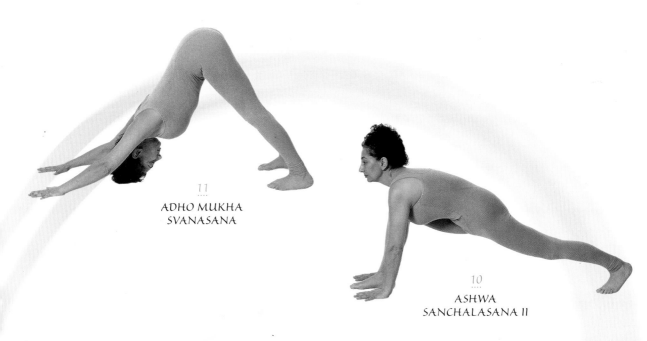

11
ADHO MUKHA
SVANASANA

10
ASHWA
SANCHALASANA II

…free the breath, free the mind
expand into consciousness

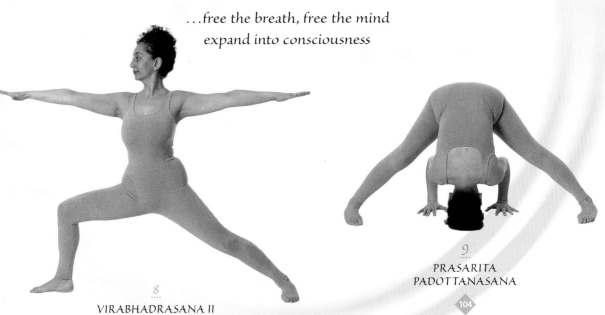

8
VIRABHADRASANA II

9
PRASARITA
PADOTTANASANA

104

◆ see FOCUS ON FLOWS section

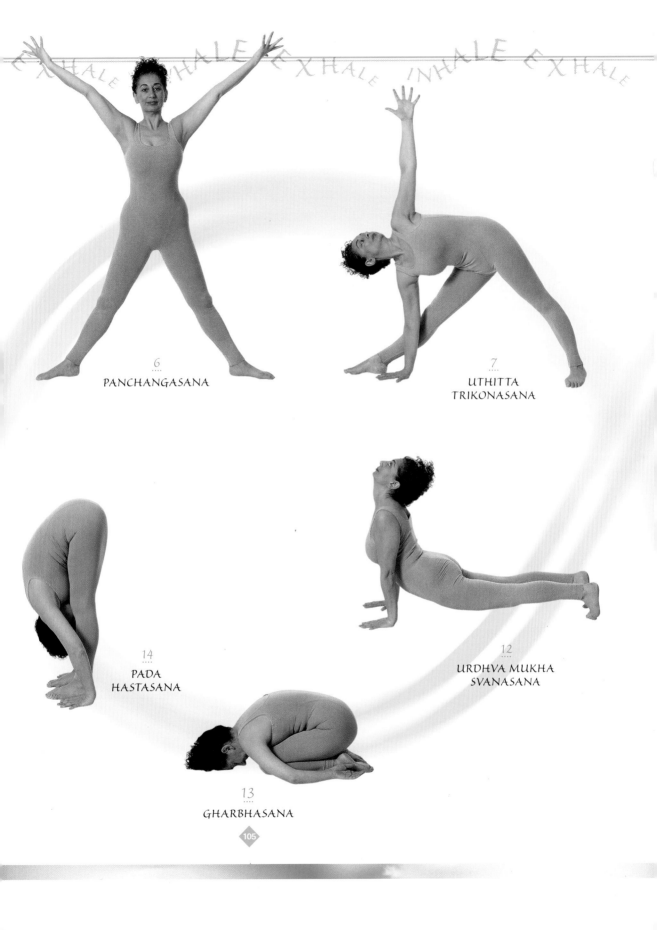

6
PANCHANGASANA

7
UTHITTA
TRIKONASANA

14
PADA
HASTASANA

12
URDHVA MUKHA
SVANASANA

13
GHARBHASANA

MAHAT YOGA PRANAYAMA
three-part breath, stage I

The complete or full yogic breath utilizes full-lung capacity to remove stale air and toxins. It enhances deep relaxation and promotes improved breathing. This increases energy production which helps renew the body's systems, creating a sense of well-being.

Breathing exercises

passive breath   Lie in *Savasana* (Corpse), your hands on your abdomen, directing the attention to your hands and watching the flow of your natural breath. Repeat, using your ribcage and clavicles, paying particular attention to each individual part.

active breath I   Repeat the above, only this time breathe in at your nostrils, paying particular attention to each of the following body parts: your abdomen (a), ribcage (b), and clavicles (c). Allow each section to rise at the inhale and fall at the exhale, controlling the flow of air. Repeat for 3–5 rounds at each section.

active breath II   As above, but breathe in only one-third of your breath at your abdomen (a), the second portion of it at your ribcage (b), and the remaining portion of it at your clavicles (c). Observe how each section consecutively expands. Exhale from the top down, pressing your navel toward your spine to expel all stale air from your lungs. Repeat for 3–5 rounds.

active breath III   Breathe in and out with all three parts simultaneously. At the very end of the exhalation, gently pull in your abdominal muscles to maximize the exhale. Repeat for 3–5 rounds.

1 Inhale. Exhaling, sit in *VAJRASANA* (Thunderbolt).

2 Inhale. Exhaling, lift up your arms in *URDHVA VAJRASANA* (Upward Thunderbolt).

3 Inhale. Exhaling, lower your torso and your arms. Rest your torso on your thighs with your arms stretched out on the ground, beyond your head, in *DHARMIKASANA* (Hare/Extended Child).

4 Inhaling, come up onto your hands and knees in Majariasana (Table). Exhale. Inhaling, keeping your toes tucked, move forward to take the weight of your body into your hands and toes. Exhaling, lower your pelvis toward the ground in *URDHVA MUKHA SVANASANA* (Upward-Facing Dog).

5 Inhale. Exhaling, lift up your tailbone, rotating your pelvis forward and upward, your head framed by your arms in *ADHO MUKHA SVANASANA* (Downward-Facing Dog).

6 Inhale. Exhaling, come down onto your hands and knees in *MAJARIASANA* (Table).

7 Inhaling, lift up your right hand. Exhaling, thread your right arm through the space between your left arm and your left knee. Place the back of your right shoulder (rather than your shoulder joint) and the back of your head on the ground in *SUTRA HASTA MAJARIASANA I* (Threading-the-Needle I).

8 Inhale. Exhaling, extend your left leg back behind your body, toes pointed. Inhale. Exhaling, lift your left arm up and back, allowing gravity to bring it down in *SUTRA HASTA MAJARIASANA II* (Threading-the-Needle II). Both your shoulders may eventually reach the ground.

9 Inhaling, carefully leave this pose by slowly taking back your arm, allowing your body to come back, and placing both hands on the ground in *MAJARIASANA* (Table).

10 Inhale. Exhaling, draw your right knee up under your chest, rest your shin on the ground and sit down behind your right heel as your body turns to face over your left leg. Inhaling, raise your arms up alongside your ears in *JANU SIRSHASANA I* (Head-to-Knee I).

11 Inhale. Exhaling, fold your body over your left leg. If your head does not reach your knee, bend your knee to meet your forehead in *JANU SIRSHASANA II* (Head-to-Knee II).

12 Inhaling, lift your head and torso. Take your right arm out horizontally and follow it with your eyes. Exhaling, place your right hand on the ground. Inhale. Look back to your left hand. Exhaling, lift your left arm out horizontally in front of you and follow it with your eyes.

Place your arm alongside your head and look up beyond your fingers. Press your right hand and shin into the ground as you lift your buttocks off the ground in *ARDHA MANDALASANA I* (Half-Circle I).

13 Inhale. Exhaling, bring your left arm down to the left as your left knee folds in to meet your right knee. Sit on your heels in Vajrasana (Thunderbolt). Inhaling, reach your arms around horizontally through the space in front of you. Exhaling, interlock your fingers behind your back and press your hands down towards your heels. Inhaling, lift your chin. Exhaling, move your torso and head forward, toward your thighs, lifting your arms up from your back as far as they can reach in *YOGA MUDRA II* (Seal of Yoga II).

14 Inhale. Exhaling, roll up onto the top of your head, lifting your buttocks away from your heels. You will feel some pressure through the crown of your head. Stabilize this by pressing equally into your knees in *YOGA MUDRA III* (Seal of Yoga III). Inhale. Exhaling, return to Yoga Mudra II (Seal of Yoga II). Inhaling, lift up your chin as you allow your arms to pull your body upward and your torso rises. Keep your heart open and your back vertical as your hands reach down to your heels on the exhale. Repeat the whole yogaflow sequence on your other side.

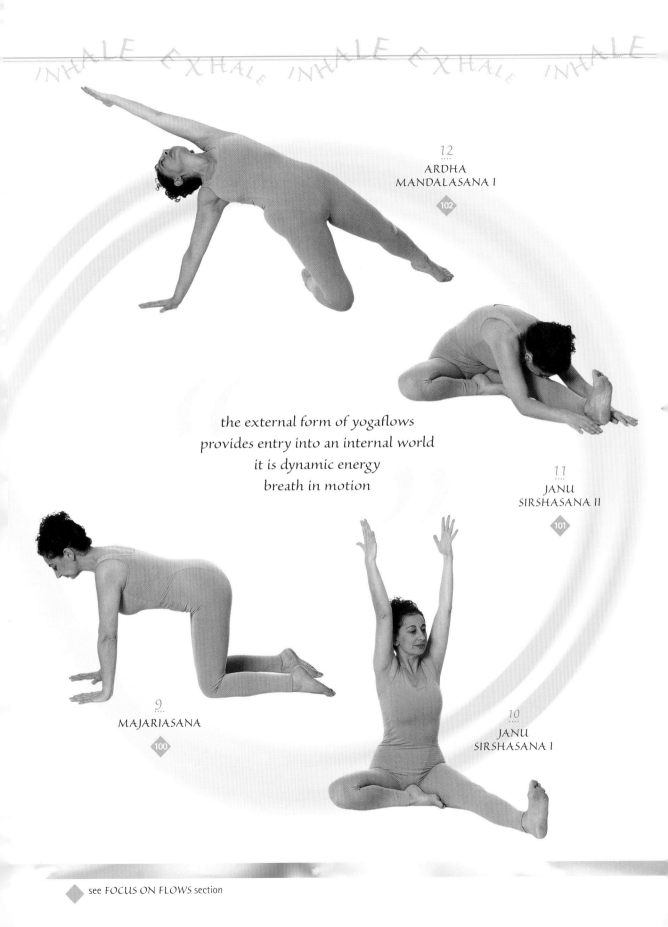

12
....
ARDHA
MANDALASANA I

102

11
....
JANU
SIRSHASANA II

101

the external form of yogaflows
provides entry into an internal world
it is dynamic energy
breath in motion

9.
....
MAJARIASANA

100

10
....
JANU
SIRSHASANA I

see FOCUS ON FLOWS section

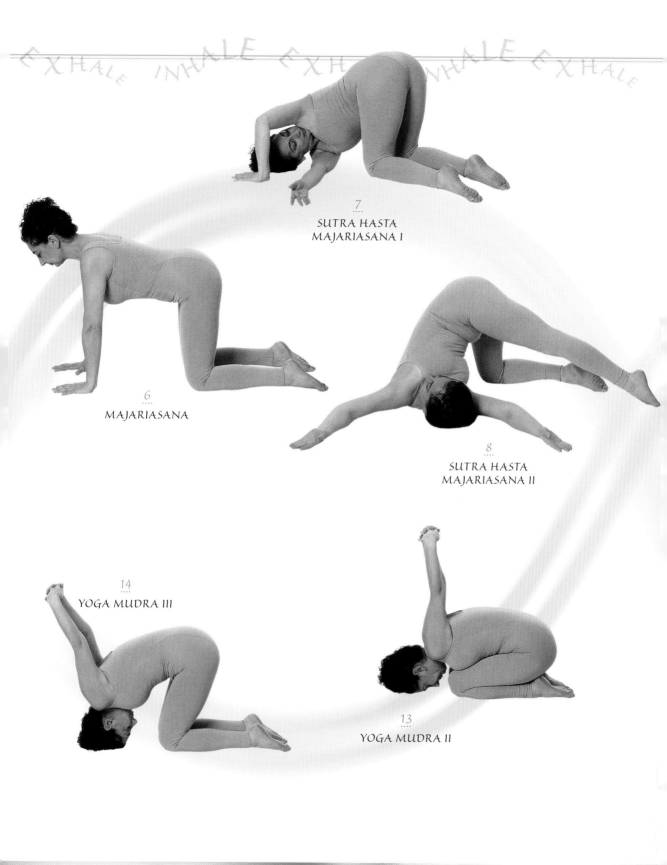

7
SUTRA HASTA
MAJARIASANA I

6
MAJARIASANA

8
SUTRA HASTA
MAJARIASANA II

14
YOGA MUDRA III

13
YOGA MUDRA II

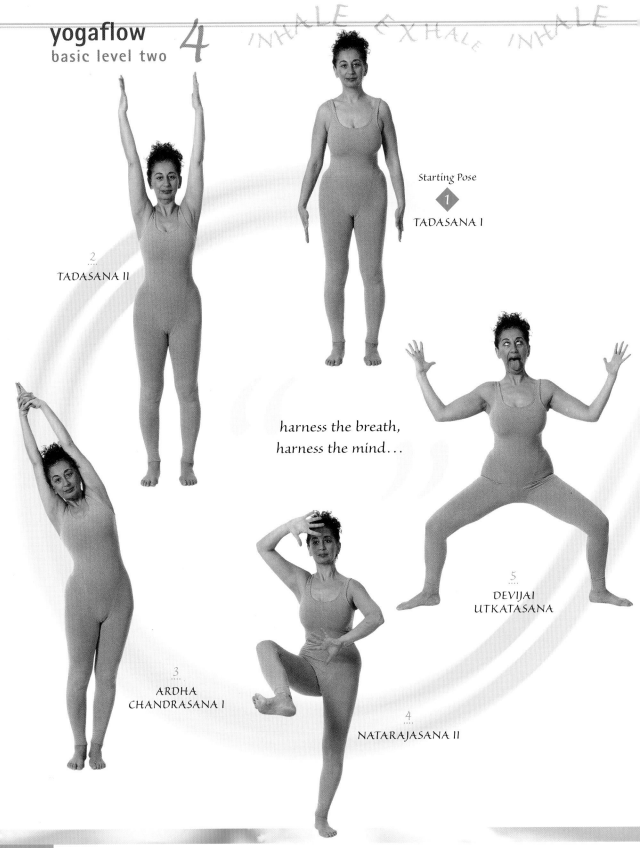

yogaflow
basic level two

4

Starting Pose

1

TADASANA I

2

TADASANA II

harness the breath,
harness the mind…

5

DEVIJAI
UTKATASANA

3

ARDHA
CHANDRASANA I

4

NATARAJASANA II

FIRE OR "HA" BREATH

This simple yet highly detoxifying, healing and stimulating practice is a distant cousin to *kapalabhathi* (shining skull breath; *see page 93*) which is a *kriya* (cleansing action), as well as a *pranayama* (breath control). Fire or "ha" breath emphasizes a forceful exhalation accompanied by a natural inhalation. Within this system, "ha" breath is used in conjunction with the dynamic warm-up practices of the book. In addition to detoxifying your body, "ha" breath massages your lungs, diaphragm, heart and abdominal organs. It cleanses, tones and purifies the many *nadis* (nerve channels) of your nervous system.

How to begin
On the exhale, allow your navel and abdominal muscles to be strongly pulled in towards your spine as your breath is forcefully expelled through your mouth to the sound of "ha". The inhale is automatic: observe how the action of your abdominal muscles and diaphragm occurs quite naturally for the inhalation. Placing a hand on your abdomen may initially help you to tune in to this area.

Notes
As the frontal parts of your brain are stimulated by this practice, dizziness, tingling and headiness may occur. If this happens, stop and breathe normally until symptoms cease. Refrain from this practice if you suffer from hyper/hypotension, have a heart condition, or are either pregnant or menstruating. Where "ha" breath is indicated, use *Ujjayi* breath instead.

As your Fire or "ha" breath practice develops and improves, make sure you do the following to prevent discomfort:

♦ *only involve your abdominal muscles;*
♦ *hold your chest still and restrict movement to your abdomen to prevent hyperventilation.*

PRANAYAMA
the yogic art of breathing

Prana is the Sanskrit word for 'life force' or 'energy'. *Ayama* means 'lengthening', 'extending' and 'expanding'. It also means 'controlling', 'restraining' and 'stopping'. Therefore, *pranayama* conveys the art of controlling and lengthening the breath.

The Sanskrit prefix *'uj'* or *'ud'* means 'to expand' or 'to raise energy', which involves an element of power, while the word *jayi* means 'success' or 'victory'. The yogic tradition teaches that if you learn to control your breath, this enables you to exercise control over your mind.

UJJAYI PRANAYAMA (Victory or Ocean Breath)

This type of breath is performed initially through your mouth with parted lips, exhaling to the sound of "haah" (as if trying to fog up a mirror) and inhaling to the sound of "aah" (as if to draw in steam) which creates a sense of coolness and dryness at the back of your throat. Practice this. When comfortable with it, start with the exhale and breathe out to "haah". Halfway through the exhale, close your mouth and continue to exhale through your nose. Repeat the same process with the inhale: breathe in to the sound of "aah" and, halfway through the inhale, close your mouth and continue to inhale through your nose.

When your mouth closes, on both the exhale and the inhale, the sound continues internally. The sound you hear will be glottal as it passes over the vocal chords in your throat. The glottis is the opening from the pharynx into the trachea (windpipe) which remains partially closed to produce the required sound during *Ujjayi* breath.

You can feel where your glottis is located by either swallowing or modulating your speech. If the passage through which your breath is escaping is narrowed, air will begin to enter more slowly, producing an audible hissing or ocean-like sound, the same one used in whispering. By consciously narrowing the passage of your throat through which air is moving, you are able to extend and control the flow of your breath. The sound emitted needs to be smooth, uninterrupted, and of uniform quality on both the exhale and the inhale.

Benefits

Practicing *pranayama* (breath control) encourages the exhalation to be as active as the inhalation. The in- and out-breath should be of equal length to maintain a continuous rhythm without interruption.

The many benefits of practicing *pranayama* can include:

- *longer inhalation and exhalation;*
- *greater concentration and mental focus;*
- *a balanced flow of the in- and out-breath;*
- *a balance in the flow of energy channels through the psychic body;*
- *a balanced nervous system;*
- *a reduced heart rate, beneficial for those with hypertension;*
- *increased heat and energy within your body;*
- *a stronger digestive system;*
- *a reduction in anxiety.*

increasing the flow
moderate warm-ups

Moderate warm-ups are a combination of stretching, opening and hara *warm-ups, a little bit more challenging than the preceding basic warm-ups (see pages 20–23). The moderate warm-ups below focus on strengthening abdominal and back muscles. Remember to keep your navel tucked in towards your spine during practice.*

1 STICK-BOAT
Lie with your body flat on the ground, legs together, feet pointed, arms above your head, palms up. Keep your back flat as you stretch (*pose a*).

Exhaling, sit up using your abdominal muscles. Keep your arms and lower legs parallel to the ground, palms facing each other, knees bent, feet pointed. Your body forms a V-shape (*pose b*). Lower your body down to the ground. Repeat dynamically. Use "ha" breath.

2 SIT-UP I
Lie with your body flat on the ground, legs together, feet pointed. Reach your arms up above your head, hands in fists. Keep your back flat as you stretch (*pose a*).

Exhaling, sweep your arms up and forward to sit upright. Keep your back straight, resting your fists on your thighs (*pose b*) and slowly roll back down, taking your arms back overhead. Repeat dynamically. Use "ha" breath.

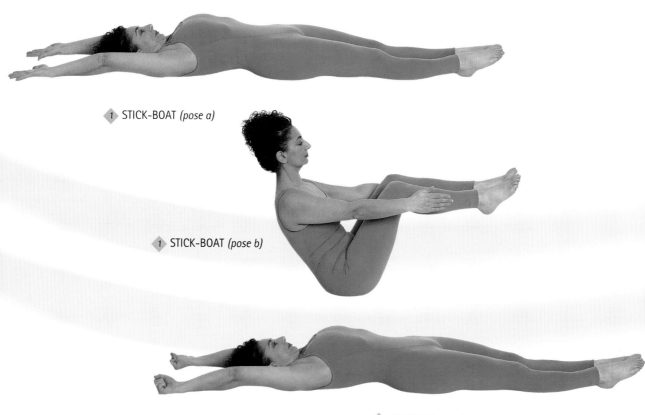

1 STICK-BOAT *(pose a)*

1 STICK-BOAT *(pose b)*

2 SIT-UP I *(pose a)*

3 SIT-UP II

Lie with your back flat on the ground, legs bent, the soles of your feet together. Reach your arms up above your head, hands in fists (*pose a*).

Exhaling, sweep your arms up and forward to sit upright. Use the strength of your abdominal muscles to bring you up (*pose b*). Slowly roll back down, taking your arms back overhead. Repeat dynamically. Use "ha" breath.

4 LEG LIFT AND VARIATIONS

Come down on all fours, knees hip-width apart, wrists beneath your shoulders, knees beneath your hips, back flat. Bring your right leg out at an angle. Lift your leg. Repeat with your left leg.

Return to starting position. Lift your right leg out at a right angle. Begin circling your right knee, directing all movement from your hip. Repeat with your left leg.

Return to starting position. Swing your right leg back as your head looks to the front. Swing your leg back and forth a few times. Repeat with your left leg. Use "ha" breath.

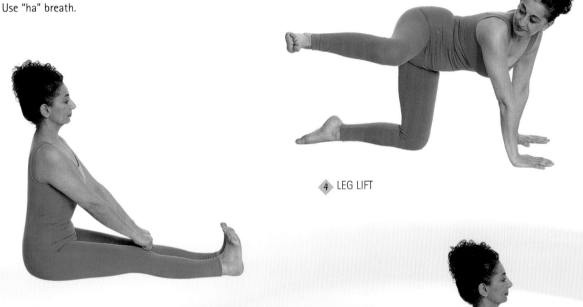

4 LEG LIFT

2 SIT-UP I *(pose b)*

3 SIT-UP II *(pose a)*

3 SIT-UP II *(pose b)*

◇5 DOLPHIN
Start on all fours, knees hip-width apart, wrists beneath your shoulders, knees beneath your hips, back flat. Lower your forearms to the ground, your elbows under your shoulders. Interlace your fingers, pressing the sides of your hands and lower arms firmly into the ground. Move your knees slightly back (*pose a*).

Tuck your toes in and press down into your arms as your knees lift, your tailbone rises, your pelvis moves up and back, your legs straighten and the soles of your feet reach toward the ground (*pose b*). Your head remains off the ground, between your arms.

Lifting your head, look up, taking your weight forward as you lower your tailbone and slightly hold your body off the ground (*pose c*). Go dynamically back and forth between the poses. Use "ha" breath.

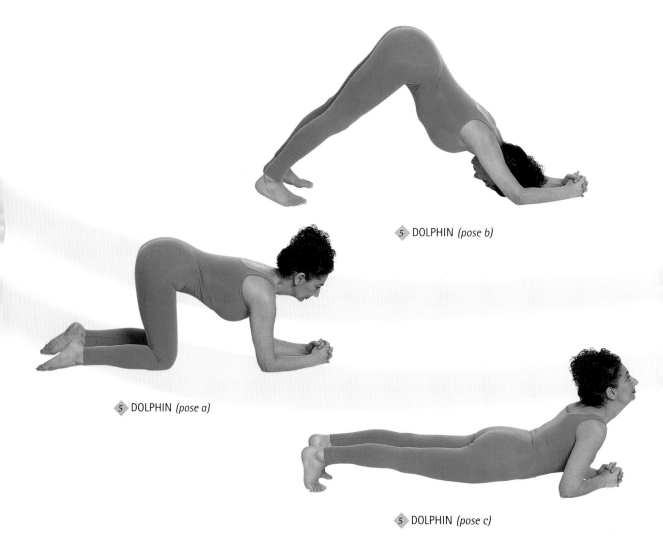

◇5 DOLPHIN (*pose b*)

◇5 DOLPHIN (*pose a*)

◇5 DOLPHIN (*pose c*)

6 ▸ TOY SOLDIER

From a sitting position with legs outstretched, lift up your arms, alongside your ears. Exhaling, lift your right leg up as your left hand comes down to touch your right toes. Keep your back straight with the crown of your head pressing upward. Return to starting position. Alternate with your left leg, gradually gathering momentum. Use "ha" breath.

7 ▸ AIRPLANE SWING

From a sitting position, spread your legs wide, keeping your back straight (sit on a block to raise your hips further, if necessary), arms out to shoulder level, feet flexed.

Exhaling, swing your body to the right from your hips with your head following your right hand. Touch your left hand to your right toes. Feel the twist in your spine. Return to starting position. Swing to the left side. Repeat dynamically, back and forth. Use "ha" breath.

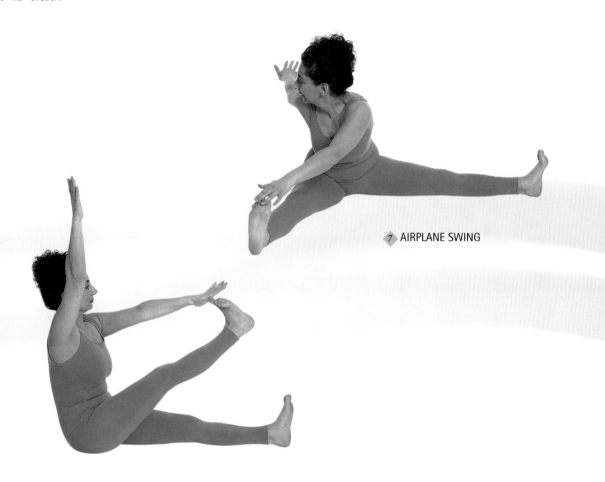

7 ▸ AIRPLANE SWING

6 ▸ TOY SOLDIER

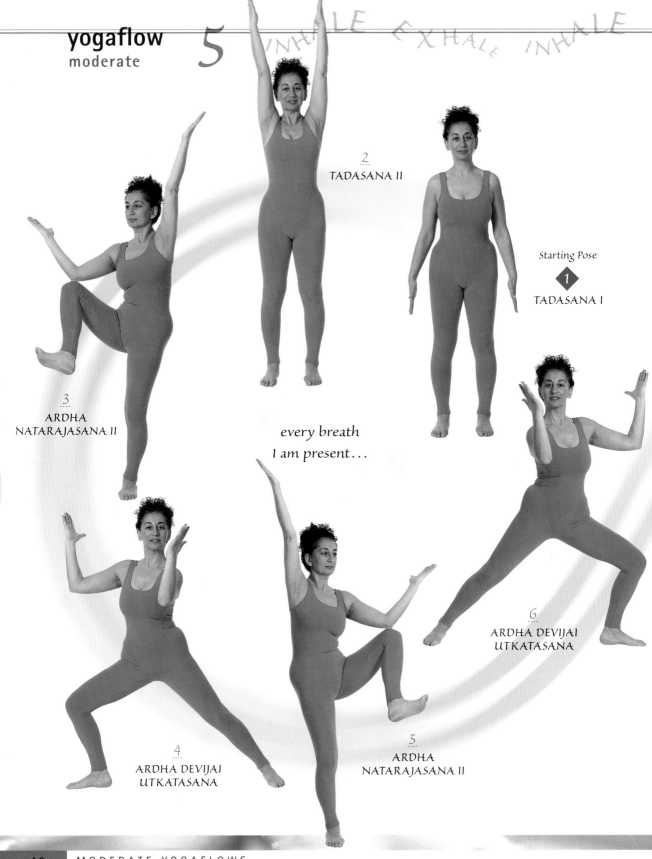

yogaflow
moderate

5

2
TADASANA II

Starting Pose
1
TADASANA I

3
ARDHA
NATARAJASANA II

*every breath
I am present…*

6
ARDHA DEVIJAI
UTKATASANA

4
ARDHA DEVIJAI
UTKATASANA

5
ARDHA
NATARAJASANA II

1 Inhale. Exhaling, start in TADASANA I (Mountain I).

2 Inhale. Exhaling, lift your arms in TADASANA II (Mountain II).

3 Inhale. Exhaling, draw your right knee toward your chest and your right elbow toward your knee in ARDHA NATARAJASANA II (Half-Dancer II, side 1).

4 Inhale. Exhaling, rotate your right arm and leg out to the right, softly landing your foot on the ground, left elbow bent, in ARDHA DEVIJAI UTKATASANA (Half-Victory Goddess Squat, side 1).

5 Inhale. Exhaling, draw your left knee toward your chest and your left elbow toward your knee in ARDHA NATARAJASANA II (Half-Dancer II, side 2).

6 Inhale. Exhaling, rotate your left arm and leg out to the left, softly landing your foot on the ground in ARDHA DEVIJAI UTKATASANA (Half-Victory Goddess Squat, side 2).

7 Inhale. Exhaling, lower into DEVIJAI UTKATASANA (Victory Goddess Squat).

8 Inhale. Exhaling, reach over to the right, keeping your right knee bent and your left leg straight. Bring your arms to shoulder level in ARDHA VIRABHADRASANA II (Half-Warrior II, side 1).

9 Inhale. Bring your body back to the center. Exhaling, reach over to the left in ARDHA VIRABHADRASANA II (Half-Warrior II, side 2). Inhale. Bring your body back to the center.

10 Inhale. Extend your right arm up alongside your head and lower your left arm to the left. Exhaling, reach upward and over to the left. Inhale. Exhaling, bend your right leg in HASTA UTTAN VIRABHADRASANA II (Warrior II Raised Arm, side 1).

11 Inhale. Repeat (10) on the other side in HASTA UTTAN VIRABHADRASANA II (Warrior II Raised Arm, side 2).

12 Inhale. Return to the right side. Exhaling, bring both arms to horizontal, turning your left foot in, right foot out, and bend your right knee to a right angle in VIRABHADRASANA II (Warrior II). Look beyond your right hand.

13 Inhale. Exhaling, rotate your left arm up and over in a circular motion. Rotate your hips to the right, squaring them over your right leg. Exhaling, move your arms down by the sides of your body. Inhale. Exhaling, raise both arms up, palms together as you look up. Inhale. Exhaling, bend your right knee to a right angle in VIRABHADRASANA I (Warrior I).

14 Inhale. Exhaling, allow your body to fold from your hips. Bring your head and arms down. Rest your hands or fingertips on the ground, either side of your right foot, your chest on your thighs. Look ahead. If possible, straighten your right leg in PARSVOTTANASANA I (Pyramid I).

15 Inhale. Exhaling, raise your body and arms back up as you rotate to the left by half-a-turn. Extend your arms up, slightly outward in a V-shape, palms facing in and back in PANCHANGASANA (Five-Pointed Star).

16 Inhale. Exhaling, lower your knees into DEVIJAI UTKATASANA (Victory Goddess Squat). Inhale. Exhaling, step your feet together and bring your arms down by your sides in Tadasana I (Mountain I). Repeat the whole yogaflow sequence on your other side.

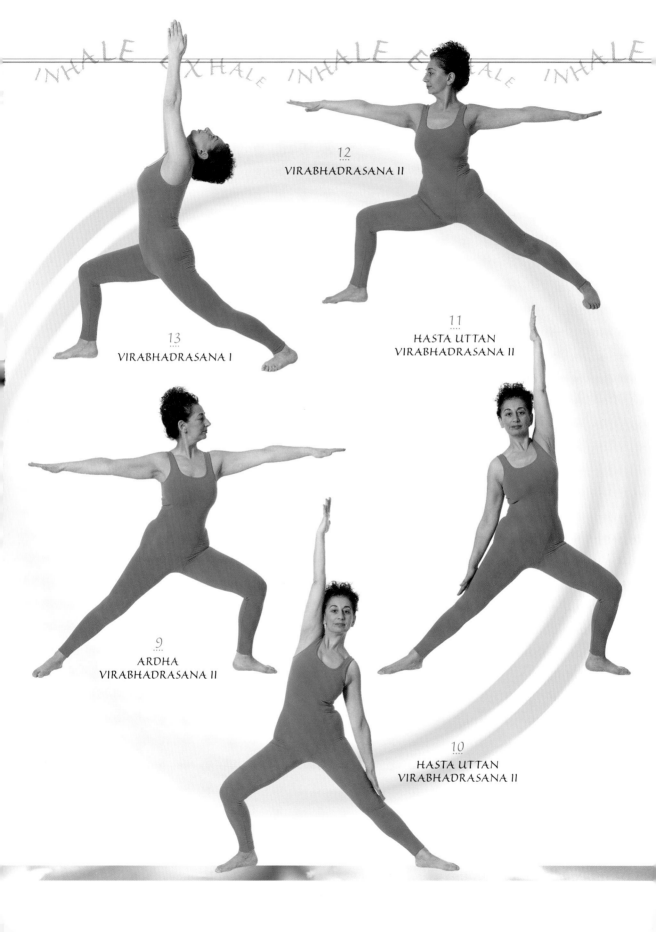

12
VIRABHADRASANA II

13
VIRABHADRASANA I

11
HASTA UTTAN
VIRABHADRASANA II

9
ARDHA
VIRABHADRASANA II

10
HASTA UTTAN
VIRABHADRASANA II

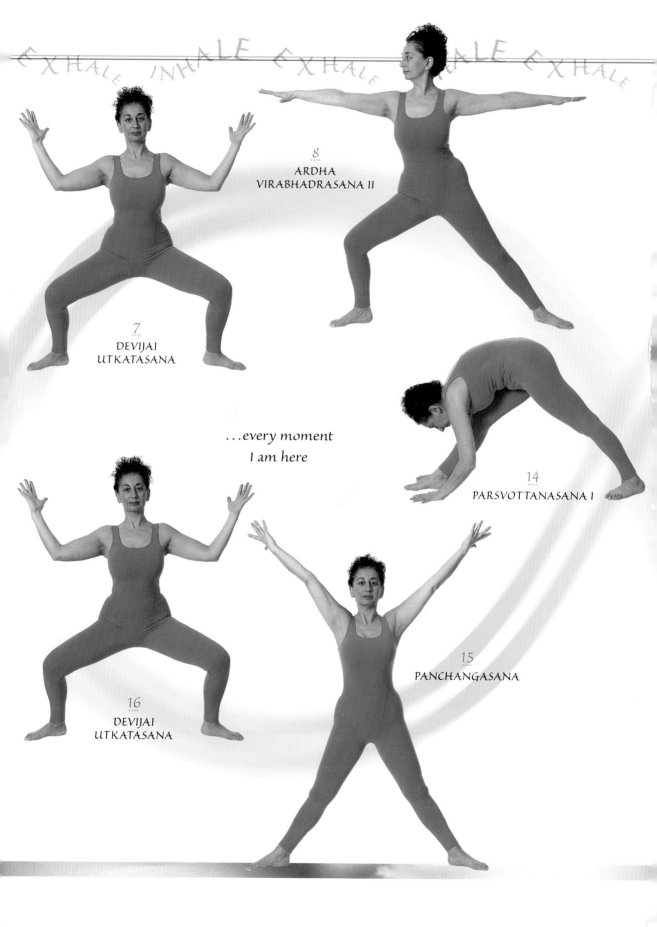

8.
ARDHA
VIRABHADRASANA II

7.
DEVIJAI
UTKATASANA

...every moment
I am here

14
PARSVOTTANASANA I

15
PANCHANGASANA

16
DEVIJAI
UTKATASANA

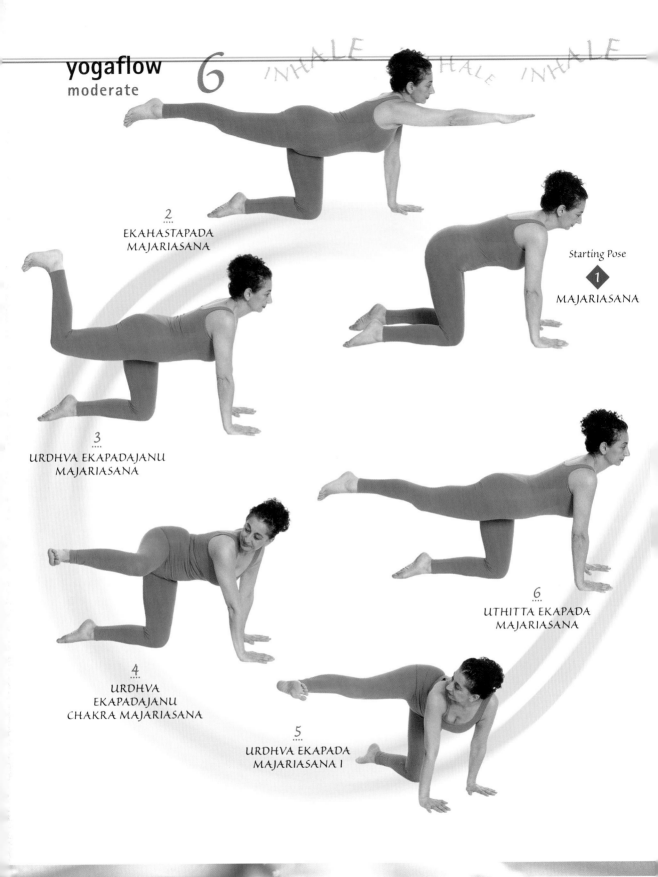

yogaflow
moderate

6

Starting Pose

1

MAJARIASANA

2

EKAHASTAPADA
MAJARIASANA

3

URDHVA EKAPADAJANU
MAJARIASANA

4

URDHVA
EKAPADAJANU
CHAKRA MAJARIASANA

5

URDHVA EKAPADA
MAJARIASANA I

6

UTHITTA EKAPADA
MAJARIASANA

1 Inhale. Exhaling, come into *MAJARIASANA* (Table).

2 Inhale. Exhaling, lift up your right arm and leg, aligning your torso, arm and leg in *EKAHASTAPADA MAJARIASANA* (One Hand-to-Foot Table Balance).

3 Inhale. Exhaling, bring your right hand back down to the ground. Inhale. Exhaling, bend your right knee, pressing the sole of your foot upward in *URDHVA EKAPADAJANU MAJARIASANA* (Upward One-Foot Hip Press).

4 Inhale. Exhaling, lift your right knee out to the side. Begin circling your leg from your hip in *URDHVA EKAPADAJANU CHAKRA MAJARIASANA* (Upward One-Foot Hip Rotation). Repeat for 5–7 rounds.

5 Inhale. Exhaling, extend your right leg out to the side. Inhaling, take your leg back in alignment with your torso. Exhaling, swing your leg to the side. Look toward the big toe of your right foot, leg parallel to the ground. Align your foot, ankle, knee and hip in *URDHVA EKAPADA MAJARIASANA I* (Upward One-Foot Leg Table I). Repeat for 5–7 rounds.

6 Inhale. Exhaling, swing your right leg back in *UTHITTA EKAPADA MAJARIASANA* (Extended One-Foot Table).

7 Inhale. Exhaling, bring your right leg out to the side in *URDHVA EKAPADA MAJARIASANA II* (Upward One-Foot Leg Table II). Look at your foot and grasp your big toe. If this is too challenging, place your foot on the ground.

8 Inhale. Exhaling, bring your head to your raised right knee in *MAJARIASANA JANU SIRSHASANA* (Table Head-to-Knee). If this is too challenging, repeat but with your foot on the ground.

9 Inhale. Exhaling, release. Inhaling, lift your leg up higher in *URDHVA EKAPADA MAJARIASANA II* (Upward One-Foot Leg Table II).

10 Inhale. Exhaling, bring your right foot down to the ground, still holding your right big toe. Sit your buttocks behind your left foot. Bring your left foot in alignment with your right inner thigh in *JANU SIRSHASANA I* (Head-to-Knee I). Inhaling, lift up your arms alongside your ears with your fingers extended.

11 Inhale. Exhaling, fold your body forward so your torso meets your thighs in *JANU SIRSHASANA II* (Head-to-Knee II).

12 Inhale. Exhaling, grasp your right big toe. Repeat (7), your left hand on the ground in *URDHVA EKAPADA MAJARIASANA II* (Upward One-Foot Leg Table II).

13 Inhale. Exhaling, bring your right leg around in front as you lower your heel to the ground. Tuck in your back toes. Inhale. Place your hands either side of your right leg or foot. Exhaling, fold your body over your right leg, foot flexed in *ARDHA PARSVOTTANASANA* (Half-Pyramid).

14 Inhale. Exhaling, move forward. Bend your right knee to a right angle, palms down, either side of your right foot. Extend your left leg and knee, pressing the back of your left knee upward. Exhaling, stretch your groin area, moving your pelvis down in *ASHWA SANCHALASANA II* (Rider's II High Lunge).

15 Inhale. Exhaling, bring down your left knee, back foot flat. Lift up your arms, palms together in *ARDHA CHANDRASANA II* (Half-Moon II).

16 Inhale. Exhaling, lower your arms and fingertips to the ground. Ground your left toes in *ASHWA SANCHALASANA I* (Rider's I Lunge).

17 Inhale. Exhaling, lift up your left knee and raise your tailbone. Step your right foot back in *ADHO MUKHA SVANASANA* (Downward-Facing Dog).

18 Inhale. Exhaling, move into *URDHVA MUKHA SVANASANA* (Upward-Facing Dog).

19 Inhale. Exhaling, release. Rest in *GHARBHASANA* (Child). Repeat the whole yogaflow sequence on your other side.

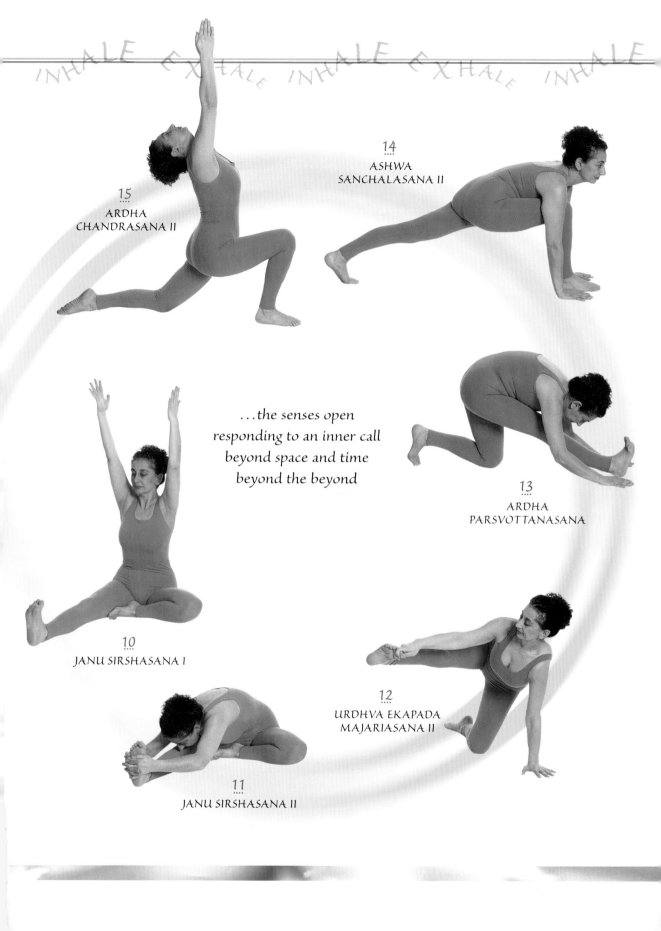

15
ARDHA
CHANDRASANA II

14
ASHWA
SANCHALASANA II

...the senses open
responding to an inner call
beyond space and time
beyond the beyond

13
ARDHA
PARSVOTTANASANA

10
JANU SIRSHASANA I

12
URDHVA EKAPADA
MAJARIASANA II

11
JANU SIRSHASANA II

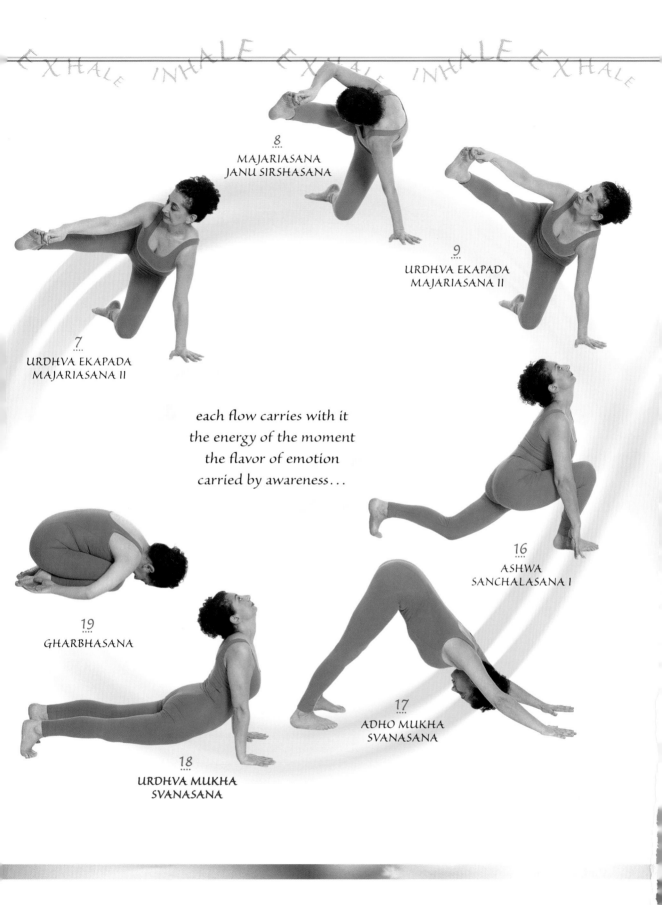

<u>8</u>

MAJARIASANA
JANU SIRSHASANA

<u>9</u>

URDHVA EKAPADA
MAJARIASANA II

<u>7</u>

URDHVA EKAPADA
MAJARIASANA II

each flow carries with it
the energy of the moment
the flavor of emotion
carried by awareness…

<u>16</u>

ASHWA
SANCHALASANA I

<u>19</u>

GHARBHASANA

<u>17</u>

ADHO MUKHA
SVANASANA

<u>18</u>

URDHVA MUKHA
SVANASANA

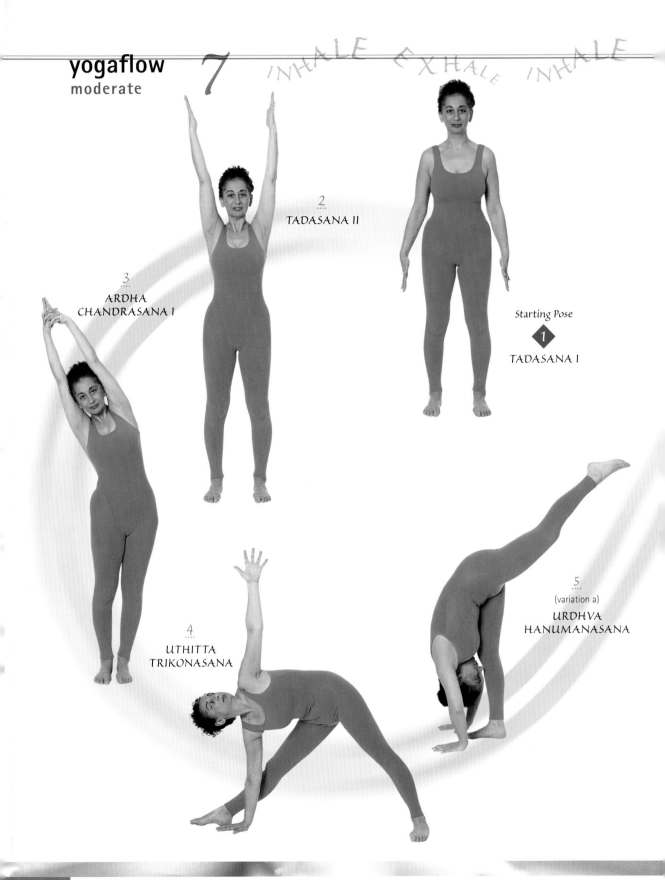

yogaflow
moderate

7

2
.....
TADASANA II

3
.....
ARDHA
CHANDRASANA I

Starting Pose

1

TADASANA I

4
.....
UTHITTA
TRIKONASANA

5
.....
(variation a)

URDHVA
HANUMANASANA

1 Inhale. Exhaling, stand in *TADASANA I* (Mountain I).

2 Inhale. Exhaling, raise your arms in *TADASANA II* (Mountain II).

3 Inhale. Exhaling, bring your feet in closer, interlock your fingers, index fingers up, thumbs crossed. Inhale. Exhaling, press your left hip and foot into the ground. Lean your body over to the right in *ARDHA CHANDRASANA I* (Half-Moon I).

4 Inhale. Return to Tadasana II (Mountain II). Exhaling, step your right leg out to the right, arms horizontal. Left foot in, right foot out. Inhale. Exhaling, reach over, tilting down to the right, right hand to the ground (foot, ankle, shin or thigh). Reach up with your left arm. Look beyond your left fingers in *UTHITTA TRIKONASANA* (Extended Triangle).

5 Inhale. Rotate your left arm back. Pivot your body and left foot in the same direction as your right foot, bending your right knee to a right angle. Touch the ground, either side of your right foot. Inhale. Exhaling, bring your chest to your right thigh as your back foot draws in toward your right foot and your palms move outward. Create a triangle with your foot and hands. Inhale. Exhaling, press your palms and right foot into the ground and lift your left leg up as high as you can, keeping your chest and thighs connected. Straighten your right leg, bringing your head toward your right knee

(a). For a more intense stretch, take your right hand to clasp your right heel, balancing on your right foot and left hand in *URDHVA HANUMANASANA* (Upward-Standing Splits). If this is too challenging, bend your right leg to a slight angle, keeping your chest and thigh connected, as you lift your back leg to just above horizontal (b). For a more basic stretch, still keeping your right knee bent into your chest, lift your left leg to just below horizontal (c).

6 Inhale. Exhaling, bring your left foot down to the ground. Inhale. Exhaling, step back into *ADHO MUKHA SVANASANA* (Downward-Facing Dog).

7 Inhale. Exhaling, keep your arms straight and come up into *URDHVA MUKHA SVANASANA* (Upward-Facing Dog).

8 Inhale. Exhaling, lower your body down, keeping your feet flat and your elbows bent. Bring your head down and come up into *BHUJANGASANA* (Cobra).

9 Exhaling, lower your body into *ADVASANA* (Reversed Corpse).

10 Inhale. Exhaling, circle your arms behind your body, lifting your torso and legs and catching your ankles. Lift into *DHANURASANA* (Bow).

11 Inhale. Exhaling, lower your body to the ground. Come into *GHARBHASANA* (Child).

12 Inhale. Exhaling, sit up on your heels in a kneeling position. Inhale. Exhaling, catch your right heel with your right hand. Inhale. Exhaling, catch your left heel with your left hand in *USHTRASANA* (Camel). To release, exhaling, take your right hand to the back right side of your pelvis first. Inhale. Then, exhaling, do the same with your left hand. Inhale. Exhaling, press your body upward. Support your back with your hands. Come to an upright position.

13 Inhale. Exhaling, come into *MAJARIASANA* (Table). Inhale. Exhaling, press your palms down, bringing your navel to your spine in Cat Tilt.

14 Inhale. Exhaling, come into *ADHO MUKHA SVANASANA* (Downward-Facing Dog).

15 Inhale. Exhaling, walk your feet toward your hands, coming into *PADA HASTASANA* (Standing Hand-to-Foot Forward Fold).

16 Inhale. Exhaling, place your right hand over your right foot, fingers facing inward, keeping your tailbone high. Exhaling, lift your right foot in your right hand, your heel toward your right buttock. Inhale. Reach out your left arm, fingers in Gyan Mudra (Seal of Knowledge). Exhaling, lift your body, extending your right leg back, away from your buttock in *NATARAJASANA I* (Dancer I). Return to Tadasana I (Mountain I). Repeat the whole yogaflow sequence on your other side.

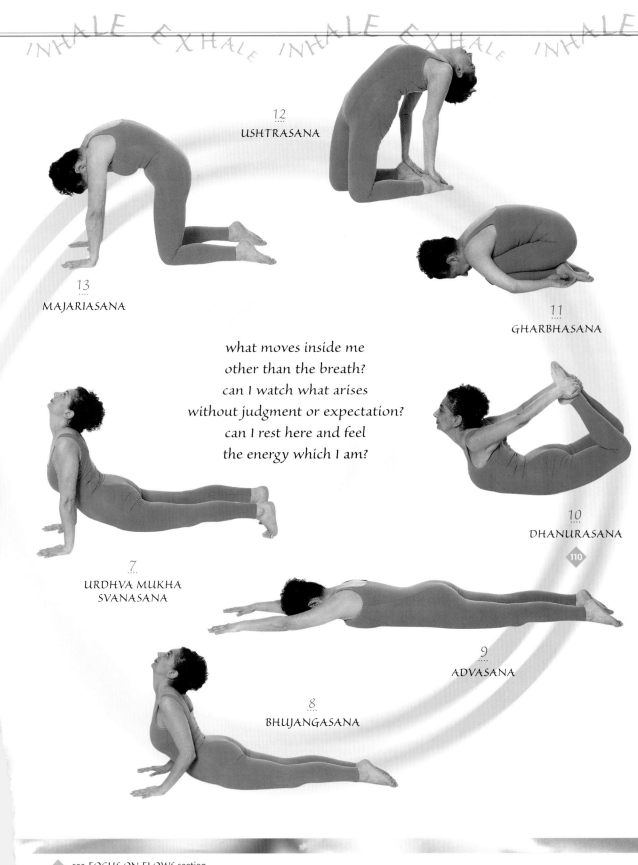

12
USHTRASANA

13
MAJARIASANA

11
GHARBHASANA

what moves inside me
other than the breath?
can I watch what arises
without judgment or expectation?
can I rest here and feel
the energy which I am?

10
DHANURASANA

110

7
URDHVA MUKHA
SVANASANA

9
ADVASANA

8
BHUJANGASANA

see FOCUS ON FLOWS section

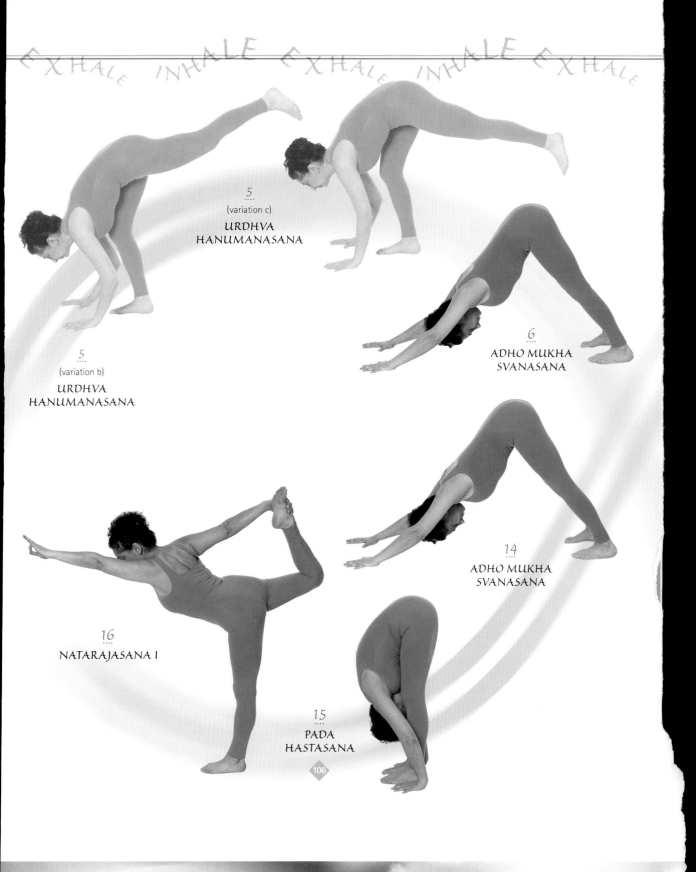

5
(variation c)

**URDHVA
HANUMANASANA**

5
(variation b)

**URDHVA
HANUMANASANA**

6

**ADHO MUKHA
SVANASANA**

14

**ADHO MUKHA
SVANASANA**

16

NATARAJASANA I

15

**PADA
HASTASANA**

8

INHALE EXHALE INHALE

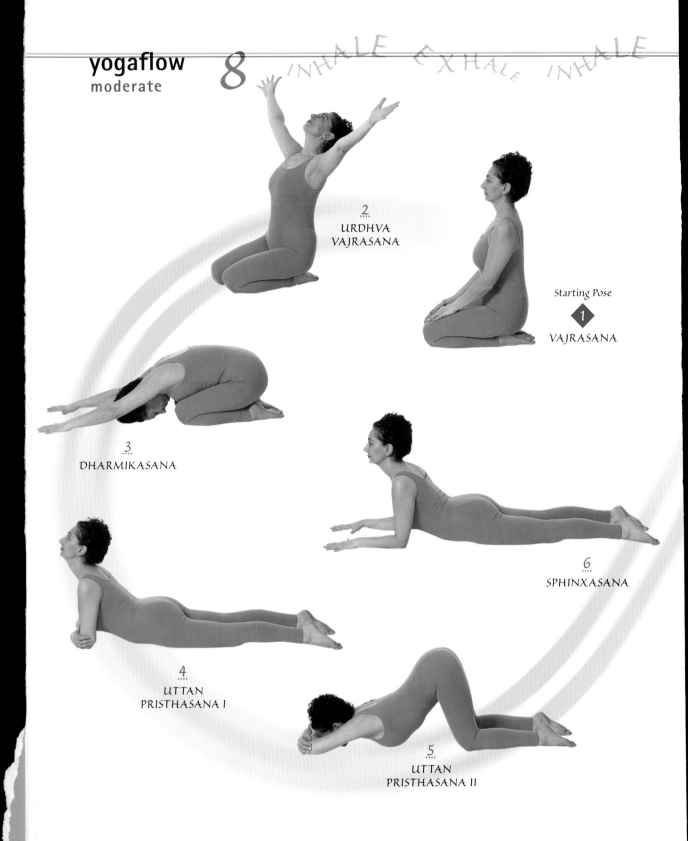

2
...
URDHVA
VAJRASANA

Starting Pose

1

VAJRASANA

3
...
DHARMIKASANA

6
...
SPHINXASANA

4
...
UTTAN
PRISTHASANA I

5
...
UTTAN
PRISTHASANA II

compassionate heart

1 Inhale. Exhaling, start in
VAJRASANA (Thunderbolt).

2 Inhale. Exhaling, raise your arms
up in URDHVA VAJRASANA
(Upward Thunderbolt).

3 Inhale. Exhaling, move into
DHARMIKASANA
(Hare/Extended Child).

4 Inhale. Lift your head, hold your
elbows, toes extended. Slide your
legs and body back in UTTAN
PRISTHASANA I (Lizard I).

5 Inhale. Exhaling, move your
tailbone up and back. Lower your
chest and chin to the ground,
flowing into UTTAN
PRISTHASANA II (Lizard II).

6 Inhale. Exhaling, release your
elbows and move your body into
SPHINXASANA (Sphinx).

7 Inhale. Keep your hands
aligned with your chest. Exhaling,
bend your right leg. Come into
KAPOTASANA (Pigeon).

8 Inhale. Exhaling, slowly allow
your body to fold forward, your
arms stretched out in front, and
your forehead on the ground in
SUPTA KAPOTASANA
(Supine Pigeon).

9 Inhale. Keep your forehead
on the ground and your chest
on your thighs. Bring your hands
back, either side of your right knee.
Tuck the toes of your left foot.
Exhaling, raise your torso in
PARSVOTTANASANA I
(Pyramid I), feet facing forward.

10 Inhaling, move your hands in
front of your right foot. Exhaling,
raise your left leg up high, keeping
your chest and thighs connected, in
URDHVA HANUMANASANA
(Upward-Standing Splits).

11 Inhale. Exhaling, bring your left
leg out to a right angle on the
ground, foot flexed, as your body
comes into JANU SIRSHASANA I
(Head-to-Knee I).

12 Inhale. Exhaling, lower
into JANU SIRSHASANA II
(Head-to-Knee II).

13 Inhale. Lift your head and flow
into ARDHA MANDALASANA I
(Half-Circle I).

14 Inhale. Lift your left leg up.
Exhaling, lower your left arm,
moving it behind your back
to hold your waist or thigh in
ARDHA MANDALASANA II
(Half-Circle II). Turn your head.
Look down.

15 Inhale. Bring your left foot
around to the outside of your right
knee. Raise your right arm in
ARDHA MATSYENDRASANA I
(Half-Spinal Twist I).

16 Inhale. Exhaling, move into
ARDHA MATSYENDRASANA II
(Half-Spinal Twist II).

17 Inhale. Exhaling, rotate your
body by half-a-turn, pressing your
hands into the ground. Come into
Vajrasana (Thunderbolt), then
YOGA MUDRA I (Seal of Yoga I).

18 Inhale. Lift your arms away
from your back as your chest moves
forward onto your thighs and your
forehead comes to the ground in
YOGA MUDRA II (Seal of Yoga II).

19 Inhale. Exhaling, lift your
buttocks up from your heels and roll
up onto the top of your head in
YOGA MUDRA III (Seal of Yoga III).

20 Inhale, carefully extend
your right leg back, stretching
it out behind you, your feet pointed
with the tops of your feet on the
ground in YOGA MUDRA IV
(Seal of Yoga IV). Inhale.
Exhaling, return back through to
Yoga Mudra III (Seal of Yoga III),
then Yoga Mudra II (Seal of Yoga II),
then Yoga Mudra I (Seal of Yoga I).
Exhaling, return your hands to your
lap in Vajrasana (Thunderbolt) but
rest in Savasana (Corpse) first.
Repeat the whole yogaflow
sequence on your other side.

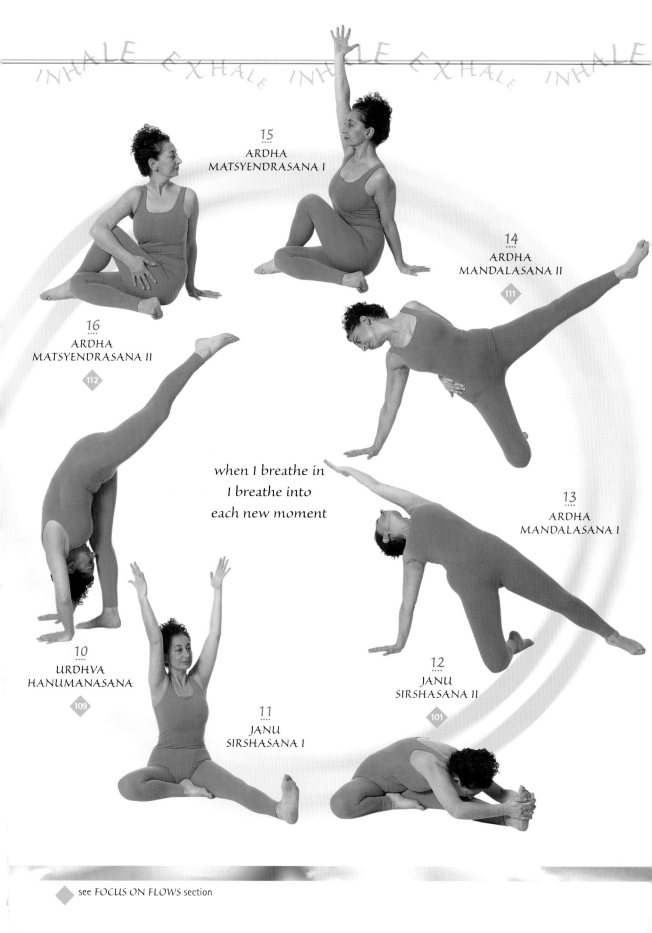

15
ARDHA
MATSYENDRASANA I

14
ARDHA
MANDALASANA II

111

16
ARDHA
MATSYENDRASANA II

112

*when I breathe in
I breathe into
each new moment*

13
ARDHA
MANDALASANA I

10
URDHVA
HANUMANASANA

109

12
JANU
SIRSHASANA II

101

11
JANU
SIRSHASANA I

see FOCUS ON FLOWS section

8
SUPTA
KAPOTASANA

108

7.
KAPOTASANA

9.
PARSVOTTANASANA I

20.
YOGA MUDRA IV

17.
YOGA MUDRA I

19.
YOGA MUDRA III

18.
YOGA MUDRA II

BANDHAS
energy body locks

Within the yogic system are practices called *bandhas*. Gathering up energy which would otherwise be dispersed, *bandhas* affect not only the physical, but also the psychic body. As a result, the endocrine and nervous systems function more efficiently, stimulating positive responses throughout your whole body. Stimulation of the root of the nervous system, which begins in the pelvic floor and ends in the crown, directly influences and modifies the way the brain receives information by balancing out mental and physical functions.

By engaging these locks through their respective physical and muscular components, energy moves in and up, flowing back into your system through your *nadis* (nerve channels) to be locked or sealed within. The benefits are not only physical: attention becomes naturally internalized, the mind is clearer, the body more grounded. By directly influencing your nervous system, *bandhas* enable you to transform stagnant energy to create heat. By maintaining these locks internally, energy is intensified and re-circulated back to tone, strengthen and nourish the physical and psychic body. Changes occur holistically and at specific cellular levels.

Types of bandhas
MOOLA BANDHA (Root or Perineum Lock)
When you start to feel comfortable in a given pose, contract the muscles between your anus and cervix (for women) and between your anus and scrotum (for men). The muscles may be difficult to locate at first and the exercise does take some practice: imagine that you want to go to the toilet and cannot find one. The muscles (both frontal and dorsal) that resist your urge to go are precisely those that you need for this exercise.

Your perineum is located between these muscles. *Moola Bandha* enhances the lift from your perineal floor into the core of your body (extending from your anus through to your crown), which encompasses all organs, blood vessels, glands and nerves. It aligns your whole skeletal structure by evenly re-distributing weight through your joints and over your feet.

UDDIYANA BANDHA (Abdominal Lock)

A full Abdominal Lock during *asana* practice is not possible as it requires your whole abdominal area to be drawn in under your ribcage on the exhale. With *Moola Bandha*, however, gentle stimulation of your lower abdomen may occur to create modified *Uddiyana Bandha* (Lower Abdominal Lock). Gently firming up the area between your hips not only stimulates the internal *agni* (fire), but also maximizes your breathing mechanism. This allows your diaphragm space to drop on the inhale by moving your ribcage during full-lung expansion. Contracting your abdominal muscles at the end of the exhale and releasing them is encouraged to fully empty out your lungs. Modified *Uddiyana Bandha* is taken up again on the next inhale. Remember not to over-expand your abdomen during inhalation, nor over-contract it during exhalation. Middle breathing is achieved through both *Moola* and *Uddiyana Bandhas*. These techniques, united with *Ujjayi* breath, represent an integral part of yoga practice, giving benefits to the mind, body and spirit.

JALANDHARA BANDHA (Chin Lock)

This practice requires you to press your chin forward, drawing it in towards the suprasternal notch in your throat after exhalation. The Chin Lock does not stop the flow of breath, but it does change it. This is not encountered too frequently during yoga poses and may occur spontaneously, for example, during *Sarvanganasana* (Shoulderstand) where the breath is not held.

freeing the flow
intensive warm-ups

Your body may be able to proceed from the previous basic and moderate exercises to these intensive warm-ups with relative ease. As you build up your practice, learn to become aware of how your body responds to each individual exercise. Alternatively, tailor-make your own exercise program, selecting various warm-ups from each of the three sections. These advanced exercises help develop physical and mental stamina, bringing renewed confidence, self-esteem and flexibility.

2 SIT-UP II
Lie with your body flat on the ground, legs together, feet flexed, arms by your sides, back flat.

Exhaling, draw your heels to your buttocks and lift your legs off the ground, thighs and shins at right angles. Lift your torso toward your knees, arms and shins parallel to the ground. Repeat dynamically.

1 SIT-UP I
Lie with your body flat on the ground, legs together, feet pointed, arms by your sides, back flat. Bend your knees and bring your legs to perpendicular. Lift your arms up overhead, palms up (*pose a*).

Exhaling, sit up, sweeping your arms up, your fingers pointing toward your feet. Keep your legs vertical (*pose b*).

Take your arms back over your head to touch the ground with the back of your hands. Keep your shoulders, head and neck off the ground. Grasp your big toes with the first two fingers of each hand, or alternatively, reach up toward your feet, gazing at your toes. Repeat dynamically. Use "ha" breath.

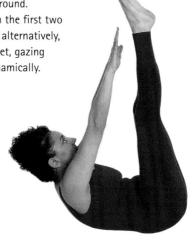

1 SIT-UP I *(pose b)*

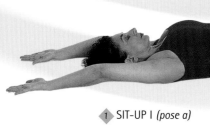

1 SIT-UP I *(pose a)*

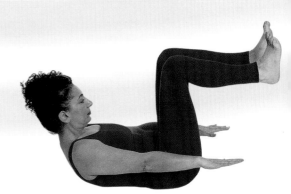

2 SIT-UP II

◆3 SIT-UP III

Lie with your body flat on the ground, legs together, feet flexed, arms by your sides, back flat. Bend your knees, extend both legs to perpendicular, lift your torso toward your legs, keeping your torso and your arms parallel to the ground. Hold.

◆4 TOY SOLDIER

From a sitting position with legs extended, feet flexed, bring your arms up, alongside your ears (*pose a*).

Exhaling, using your abdominal muscles, lift both legs up in front of you as your hands come to meet your toes in front of your eyes (*pose b*). Return to starting position. Use "ha" breath. Repeat dynamically.

◆5 HIP OPENER AND VARIATIONS

From a kneeling position, lay your torso over your thighs, forehead to the ground, arms extended in front. Lift up your buttocks, tucking your toes under, knees hip-width apart. Press into your hands and toes as your knees lift. Raise your tailbone and move your pelvis up and back. Lift your shoulders back, away from your ears, feet flat on the ground.

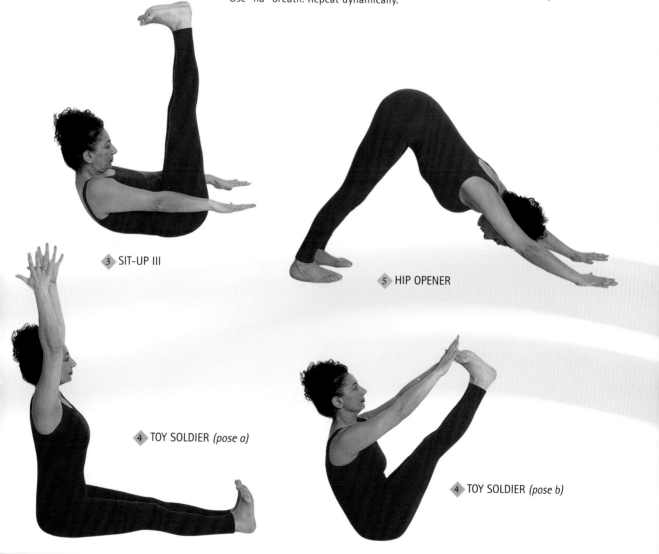

◆3 SIT-UP III

◆5 HIP OPENER

◆4 TOY SOLDIER (*pose a*)

◆4 TOY SOLDIER (*pose b*)

Bring your right leg up behind your body. Hold. Open your right hip out to the side. Bend your right knee, foot flexed. Press your right sole back as your body moves outward.

Keep pressing into your hands and stretch back through your arms. Extend your right leg outward. Begin circling your leg in one direction, then the other. Feel the action coming your hip. Lower your leg down to the ground. Hold and release.

Fold your chest and your abdomen over bent knees, forehead to the ground. Repeat using your left leg.

6 PEACOCK I

Come down on all fours, knees hip-width apart, wrists beneath your shoulders, knees beneath your hips, back flat. Rest your forearms on the ground with your elbows beneath your shoulders (pose a).

Press into your forearms as you lift your knees, raise your tailbone and move your pelvis up and back, until your feet are flat on the ground (pose b). Your head remains between your arms.

Pressing into your forearms, drop your tailbone down and lift up your head and torso (pose c). Do not lower your body too far down at first. Build this pose up in stages. Go dynamically back and forth. Use "ha" breath.

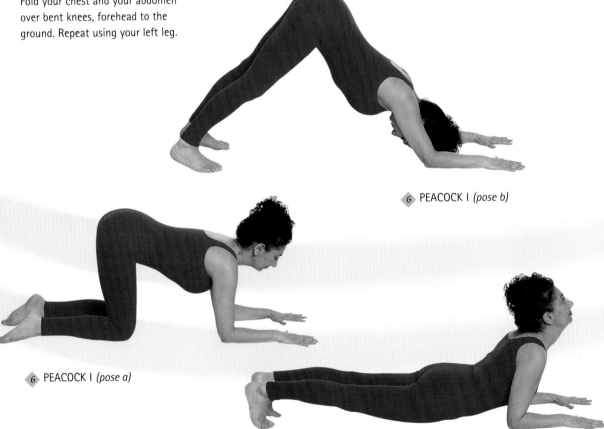

6 PEACOCK I (pose b)

6 PEACOCK I (pose a)

6 PEACOCK I (pose c)

7 PEACOCK II

Come down on all fours, knees hip-width apart, wrists beneath your shoulders, knees beneath your hips, back flat. Exhaling, raise your right leg behind your body, slightly bending your elbows (*pose a*).

Exhaling, lower your sternum down to the ground, bending your elbows toward the sides of your body. As you lower your body down, raise your right leg up behind you. Keep your elbows close to your body, pressing your hands into the ground as your chest moves slightly forward (*pose b*). Use "ha" breath. Come up. Repeat with your left leg.

8 LEG CIRCLE

Lie with your body flat on the ground, legs together, feet pointed, arms by your sides, palms up. Take your arms out to shoulder level and bring your right leg to perpendicular. Begin circling it, activating the movement from your hip.

Exhaling, cross it over your body to create a deep twist. Lift your leg up and over to the outside of your body. This is a great posture for hip-opening and release. Use "ha" breath. Repeat using your left leg.

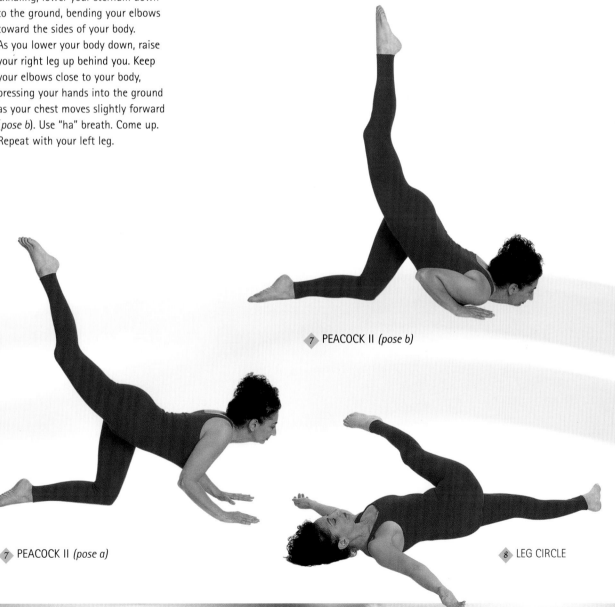

7 PEACOCK II *(pose b)*

7 PEACOCK II *(pose a)*

8 LEG CIRCLE

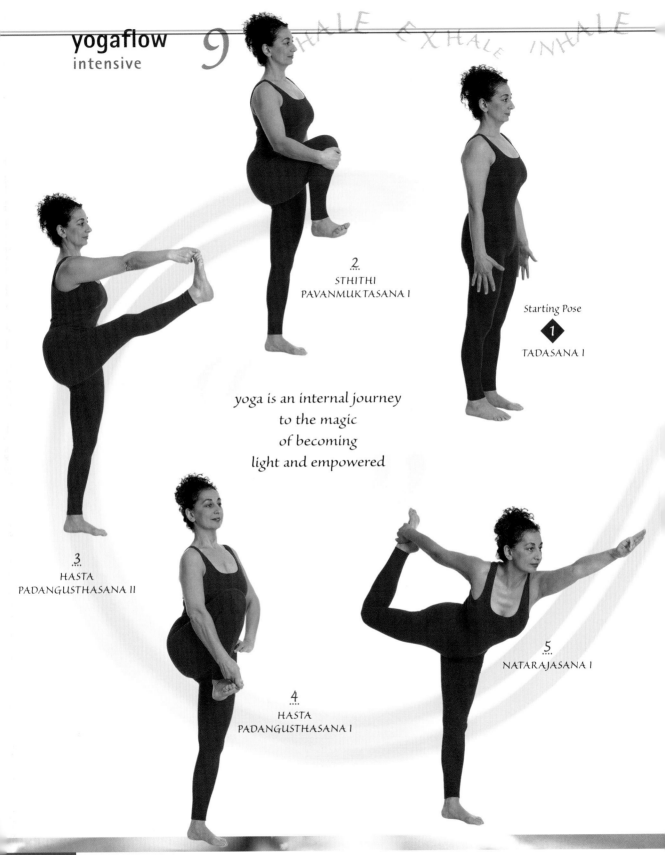

9 INHALE EXHALE INHALE

2.
STHITHI
PAVANMUKTASANA I

Starting Pose

1

TADASANA I

3.
HASTA
PADANGUSTHASANA II

yoga is an internal journey
to the magic
of becoming
light and empowered

5.
NATARAJASANA I

4.
HASTA
PADANGUSTHASANA I

1 Inhale. Exhaling, come into TADASANA I (Mountain I).

2 Inhale. Exhaling, place your left hand on your left hip and your right knee up to your chest in STHITHI PAVANMUKTASANA I (Standing Wind-Relieving I). There is an intermediary stage between poses 2 and 3. If holding your big toe as you extend your leg out to the horizontal is too challenging, keep your knee bent in toward your chest. Hold your big toe, keeping your chest upright, gradually straightening your leg.

3 Inhale. Exhaling, hook your right big toe with your thumb and the first two fingers of your right hand. Inhale. Exhaling, extend your right leg away from you in HASTA PADANGUSTHASANA II (Hand-to-Foot Big Toe II).

4 Inhale. Exhaling, still holding your right big toe, draw your knee into your chest, your right elbow on the outside of your leg in HASTA PADANGUSTHASANA I (Hand-to-Foot Big Toe I).

5 Inhale. Exhaling, place your right hand over the top of your right foot as you bring your right heel back toward your right buttock, aligning both knees. Raise your left arm in front of your body, left hand in Gyan Mudra (Seal of Knowledge). Extend your right leg back, bring your body to horizontal and look toward your fingertips in NATARAJASANA I (Dancer I).

6 Inhale. Exhaling, rotate your body back up to the center. Release your right foot, bringing it down to the ground, legs astride. Reach your right arm towards your ankle, palm down, in UTHITTA TRIKONASANA (Extended Triangle).

7 Inhale. Exhaling, come up. Rotate your ribcage to the right in PARIVRTTA UTHITTA TRIKONASANA (Revolved Extended Triangle).

8 Inhale. Exhaling, bring your body back to the center. Inhale. Exhaling, bend your right leg, placing your right hand on the outside of your right foot in PARSVAKONASANA (Lateral Angle).

9 Inhale. Exhaling, come up. Inhale. Exhaling, bring your body back to the center as your right leg straightens, feet parallel. Extend your arms behind your body, fingers interlaced. Exhaling, fold forward, lifting your arms up and away from your back in PRASARITA PADOTTANASANA YOGA MUDRA (Spread-Leg Forward Fold Seal of Yoga).

10 Inhale. Exhaling, come up. Exhaling, release your hands and lower your right knee down to the ground. Keep your left leg out to the side, toes pointing outward in PARIGHASANA I (Gate I).

11 Inhale. Exhaling, extend over into PARIGHASANA II (Gate II).

12 Inhale. Exhaling, lift up and bring your right hand to the ground and your left arm up in PARIGHASANA III (Gate III) to reverse the extension.

13 Inhale. Exhaling, rotate your left arm up and over as your body turns to face over your right knee. Inhale. Exhaling, bring your right foot and place it on your left knee as your left leg is raised off the ground. Lean your body slightly forward and balance in EKAPADA JANU MAJARIASANA (One-Foot Table Balance).

14 Inhale. Exhaling, release your right leg down to the ground. Keeping your left leg parallel to the ground, drop your body weight forward onto your hands, bending your elbows as your chest and chin are lowered to the ground. As your body weight is being lowered, lift your left leg up as high as you can in EKAPADA DANDA MAJARIASANA (One-Foot Table Press-Up).

15 Inhale. Exhaling, step back into ADHO MUKHA SVANASANA (Downward-Facing Dog).

16 Inhale. Exhaling, walk your feet toward your hands into PADA HASTASANA (Standing Hand-to-Foot Forward Fold). Exhaling, lift your body up into Tadasana I (Mountain I). Repeat the whole yogaflow sequence on your other side.

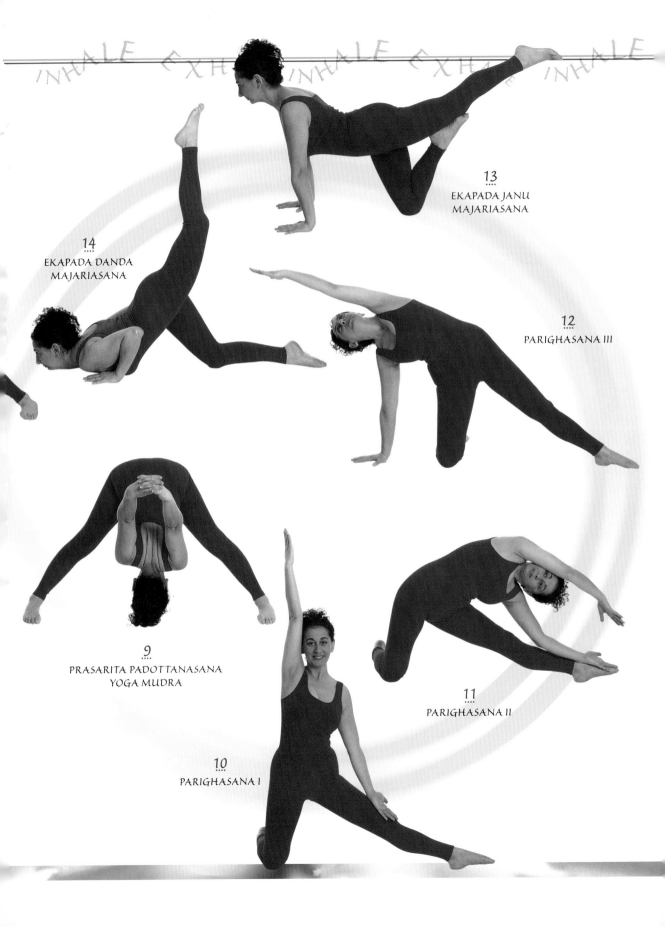

13
EKAPADA JANU
MAJARIASANA

14
EKAPADA DANDA
MAJARIASANA

12
PARIGHASANA III

9
PRASARITA PADOTTANASANA
YOGA MUDRA

11
PARIGHASANA II

10
PARIGHASANA I

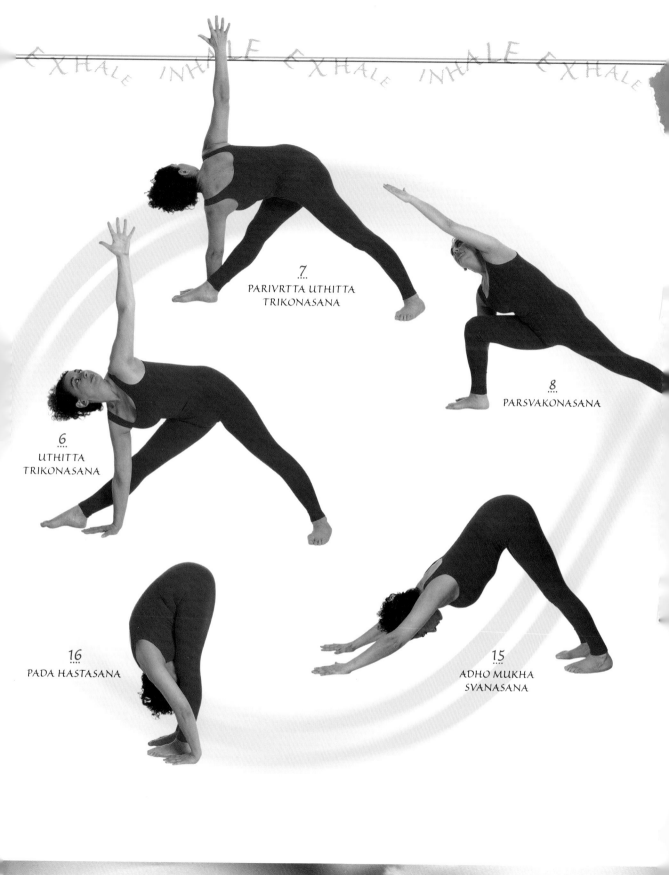

7
PARIVRTTA UTHITTA
TRIKONASANA

8
PARSVAKONASANA

6
UTHITTA
TRIKONASANA

16
PADA HASTASANA

15
ADHO MUKHA
SVANASANA

INHALE EXHALE INHALE

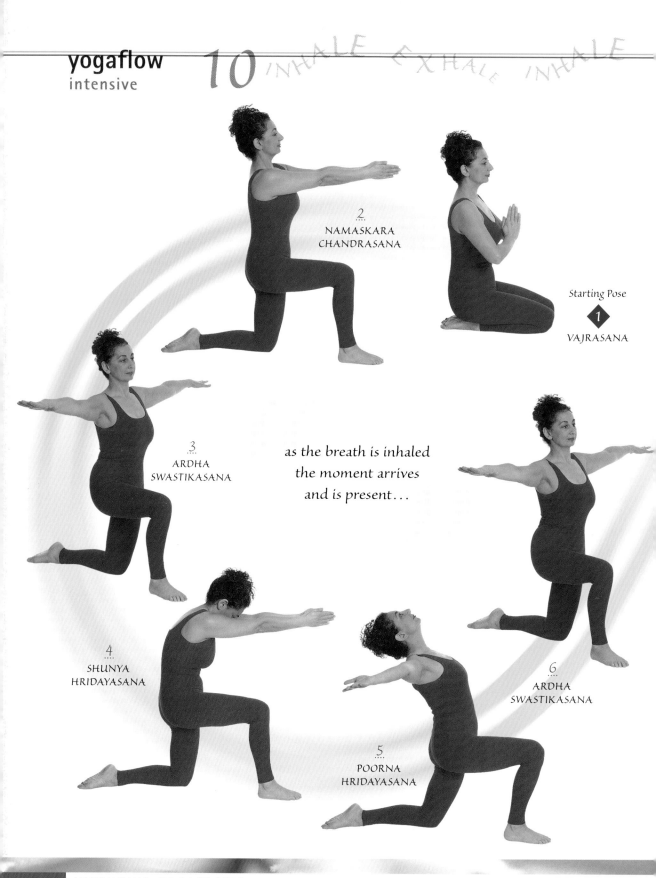

2.
NAMASKARA
CHANDRASANA

Starting Pose

1

VAJRASANA

3.
ARDHA
SWASTIKASANA

as the breath is inhaled
the moment arrives
and is present…

4.
SHUNYA
HRIDAYASANA

6.
ARDHA
SWASTIKASANA

5.
POORNA
HRIDAYASANA

Use padding for your knees when practicing this yogaflow.

1 Inhale. Exhaling, start in VAJRASANA (Thunderbolt), hands in Pranamasana (Prayer).

2 Inhaling, lift your buttocks off your heels and come onto your knees. Bring your right foot forward, at a right angle with your right knee, arms out in front, parallel to the ground, palms together in NAMASKARA CHANDRASANA (Salutation to the Moon).

3 Inhaling, open your arms out at shoulder level, palms down, in ARDHA SWASTIKASANA (Half-Cross).

4 Exhaling, press your back away from you, pelvis in Cat Tilt, as your arms come out in front of you, palms together, your head between your arms in SHUNYA HRIDAYASANA (Empty Heart).

5 Inhaling, lift your chest, pelvis in Dog Tilt, arms out, palms facing up. Lift up head and chin in POORNA HRIDAYASANA (Full Heart).

6 Exhaling, bring your upper body back to vertical. Hold your arms out at shoulder level in ARDHA SWASTIKASANA (Half-Cross).

7 Inhale. Exhaling, tilt your body down to the right, fingers touching the ground. Look beyond your left fingers. Come back. Exhaling, repeat on your left side. Look beyond your right fingers in CHANDRA KONASANA (Moon Side Angle).

8 Inhale. Exhaling, rotate to the right. Look along your right arm. Come back. Repeat on the left side in PARIVRTTA CHANDRA KONASANA (Revolved Moon Side Angle).

9 Inhale. Exhaling, tuck in the toes of your left foot. Inhaling, extend your right arm up. Touch your left heel with your left hand. Look up in ARDHA USHTRASANA CHANDRASANA (Half-Camel Moon).

10 Inhaling, extend your left arm up. Touch your left heel with your right hand. Look up in PARIVRTTA ARDHA USHTRASANA CHANDRASANA (Revolved Half-Camel Moon).

11 Inhaling, extend your right arm up. Exhaling, lift your left lower leg, clasping your left foot in your left hand, right fingers in Gyan Mudra (Seal of Knowledge). Look up in EKAPADA CHANDRA NATARAJASANA I (One-Foot Moon Dancer I).

12 Inhale. Exhaling, draw your left heel toward your buttock. Move your body forward over your right thigh in EKAPADA CHANDRA NATARAJASANA II (One-Foot Moon Dancer II).

13 Exhaling, come up. Inhale. Clasp your left foot with both hands. Exhaling, press it into your hands, straightening your arms. Move your heel away from your buttock and look up in EKAPADA CHANDRA NATARAJASANA III (One-Foot Moon Dancer III).

14 Inhale. Exhaling, move your trunk to the inside of your right thigh, your left heel toward your left buttock. Bring your head down on the inside of your right knee in EKAPADA CHANDRA NATARAJASANA IV (One-Foot Moon Dancer IV).

15 Inhaling, release your hands from your foot as your chin and chest lift up and back. Exhaling, sweep your arms down, then up into a V-shape, in ARDHA CHANDRASANA II (Half-Moon II).

16 Inhale. Exhaling, tuck your left toes in, folding your body forward. Move your hips toward your left heel. Extend your right leg, foot flexed. Rest your chest on your right thigh, head to knee, in ARDHA PARSVOTTANASANA (Half-Pyramid).

17 Inhaling, raise your buttocks. Move forward, palms flat, left leg extended, toes tucked in, back knee straight. Exhale, hips down in ASHWA SANCHALASANA II (Rider's II High Lunge).

18 Inhale. Exhaling, step your right foot back into ADHO MUKHA SVANASANA (Downward-Facing Dog). Return to Vajrasana (Thunderbolt). Repeat the whole yogaflow sequence on your other side.

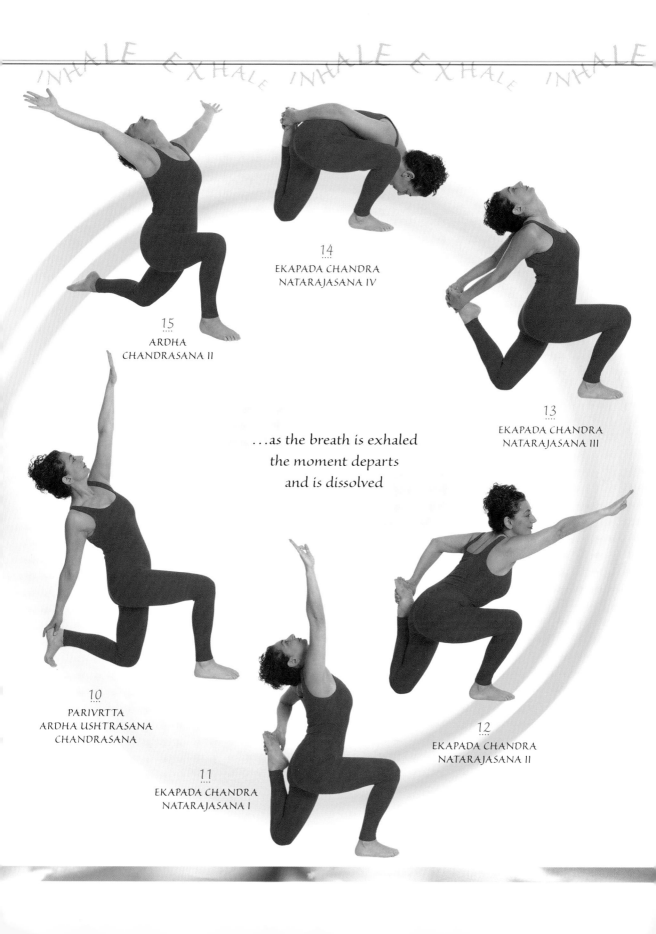

14
EKAPADA CHANDRA
NATARAJASANA IV

15
ARDHA
CHANDRASANA II

13
EKAPADA CHANDRA
NATARAJASANA III

...as the breath is exhaled
the moment departs
and is dissolved

10
PARIVRTTA
ARDHA USHTRASANA
CHANDRASANA

11
EKAPADA CHANDRA
NATARAJASANA I

12
EKAPADA CHANDRA
NATARAJASANA II

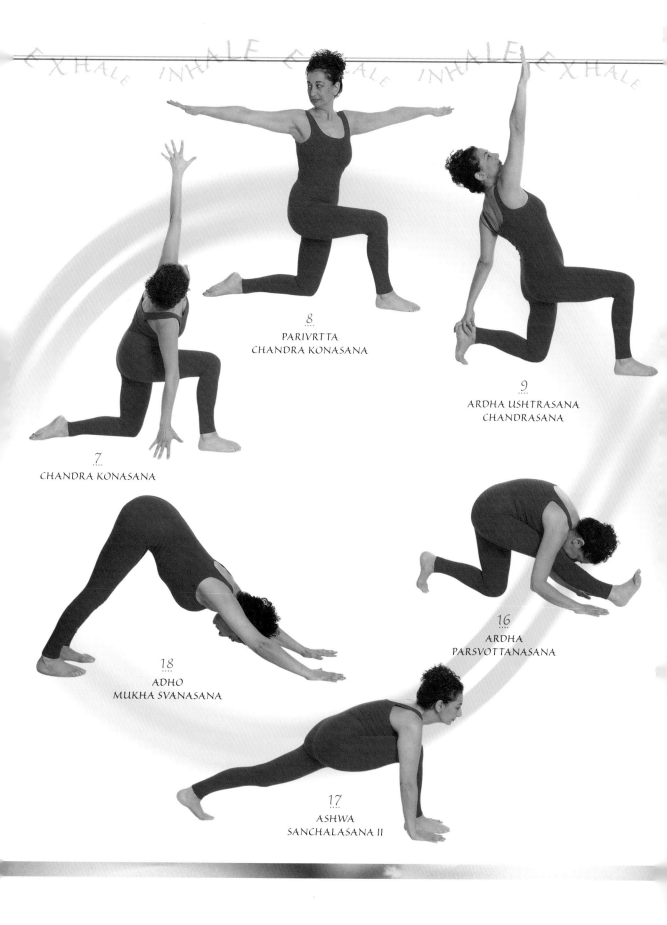

8
PARIVRTTA
CHANDRA KONASANA

9
ARDHA USHTRASANA
CHANDRASANA

7
CHANDRA KONASANA

18
ADHO
MUKHA SVANASANA

16
ARDHA
PARSVOTTANASANA

17
ASHWA
SANCHALASANA II

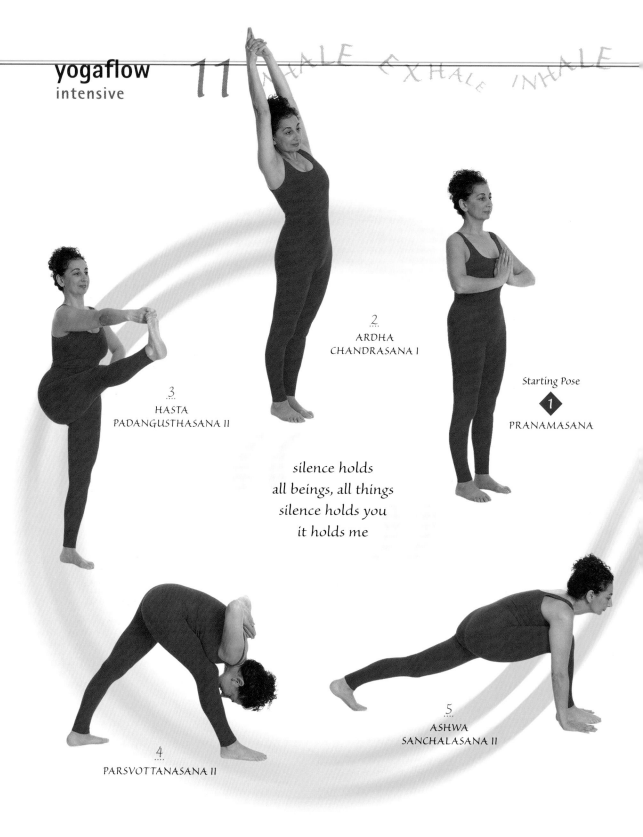

11 INHALE EXHALE INHALE

2.
ARDHA
CHANDRASANA I

3.
HASTA
PADANGUSTHASANA II

Starting Pose
1
PRANAMASANA

silence holds
all beings, all things
silence holds you
it holds me

5.
ASHWA
SANCHALASANA II

4.
PARSVOTTANASANA II

1 Inhale. Exhaling, come into PRANAMASANA (Prayer).

2 Inhaling, narrow the gap between your feet, raising your arms in ARDHA CHANDRASANA I (Half-Moon I) and exhale.

3 Inhaling, take your body back to the center. Exhaling, lower your left hand to your hip, fingers spread. Inhaling, raise your right foot, hook your big toe with your right index and second finger. Exhaling, extend your right leg to horizontal in HASTA PADANGUSTHASANA II (Hand-to-Foot Big Toe II).

4 Inhale. Exhaling, release your toe. Bend your back knee, stepping your right foot in front. Leave a wide gap between your feet, hands in Namaskara (Salutation), behind your back. Face over your forward leg, straightening both legs. Inhale. Exhaling, fold your body forward, leading with your sternum, your chest toward your thighs, in PARSVOTTANASANA II (Pyramid II).

5 Inhale. Exhaling, release your hands. Bend your right knee in ASHWA SANCHALASANA II (Rider's II High Lunge).

6 Inhaling, flatten the toes of your left foot. Exhaling, bring your left knee down, raising your arms in ARDHA CHANDRASANA II (Half-Moon II).

7 Inhale. Exhaling, lower your arms to horizontal. Twist your body to the right. Wedge your left lower arm against the outside of your right knee. Extend your right arm back and look beyond your right fingers in PARIVRTTA ARDHA CHANDRASANA (Revolved Half-Moon). Breathe freely.

8 Inhale. Exhaling, slide your left arm along your right leg, palms in Namaskara (Salutation). Look over your right shoulder in NAMASKARA PARIVRTTA PARSVAKONASANA I (Revolved Salutation Side Angle I).

9 Exhaling, rotate your trunk to the right, turning your back toes in. Lift your left knee, turn your foot in. Straighten your leg. Increase the twist in your torso by pressing your left arm deeper into your right leg in NAMASKARA PARIVRTTA PARSVAKONASANA II (Revolved Salutation Side Angle II).

10 Inhale. Exhaling, return your body back to the center, hands either side of your right foot, legs straight, torso folding forward in PARSVOTTANASANA I (Pyramid I).

11 Inhale. Exhaling, lift your left leg in URDHVA HANUMANASANA (Upward-Standing Splits).

12 Inhale. Exhaling, lower your left leg. Rotate your body to the right, feet parallel. Inhaling, with your arms behind your back, interlace your fingers. Lift up your arms as your body moves forward into PRASARITA PADOTTANASANA YOGA MUDRA (Spread-Leg Forward Fold Seal of Yoga).

13 Inhale. Exhaling, lower your arms, keeping your palms flat. Turn your feet, torso and hands to the right. Inhaling, tuck in your left toes and bring your left knee to the ground. Exhaling, take your weight back to sit on your left heel. Extend your right leg in front, placing your left hand on the ground for balance. Hold your right foot with your right hand. Exhaling, take your weight back further, flattening your left foot as you lift your right leg with your right hand. Join your left hand with your right hand, interlacing fingers around your right foot in UTTHITA EKAPADA ANGUSTHASANA (Extended One-Leg Tiptoe).

14 Inhale. Exhaling, release your right foot. Inhaling, move forward, bending your right knee. Extend your left leg back in ASHWA SANCHALASANA I (Rider's I Lunge).

15 Inhale. Exhaling, step into PADA HASTASANA (Standing Hand-to-Foot Forward Fold).

16 Inhale. Exhaling, rise to HASTA UTTANASANA (Raised Arms). Inhale. Exhaling, lower your arms to Pranamasana (Prayer). Repeat the whole yogaflow sequence on your other side.

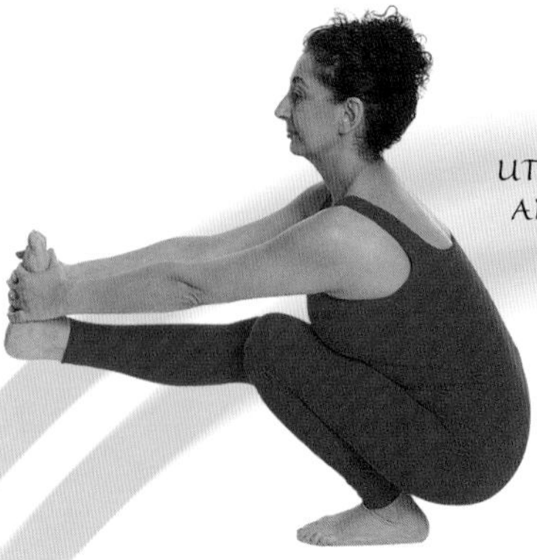

13
UTHITTA EKAPADA
ANGUSTHASANA

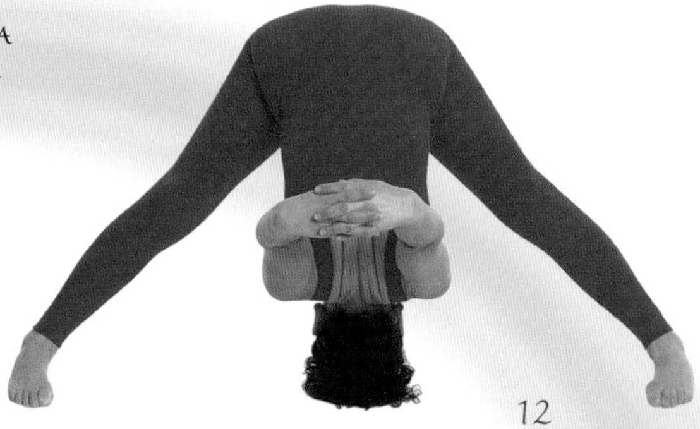

12
PRASARITA
PADOTTANASANA
YOGA MUDRA

114

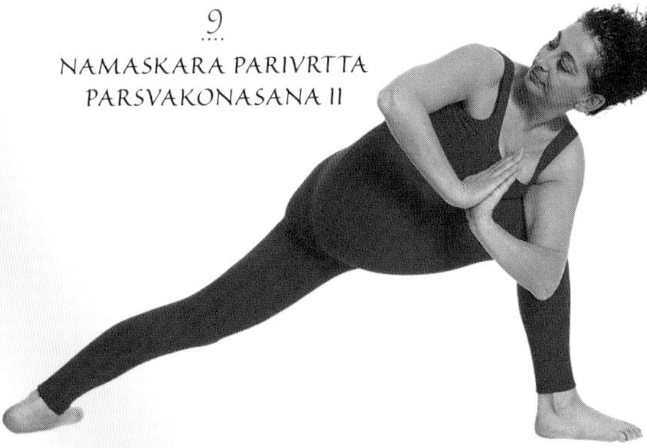

9
NAMASKARA PARIVRTTA
PARSVAKONASANA II

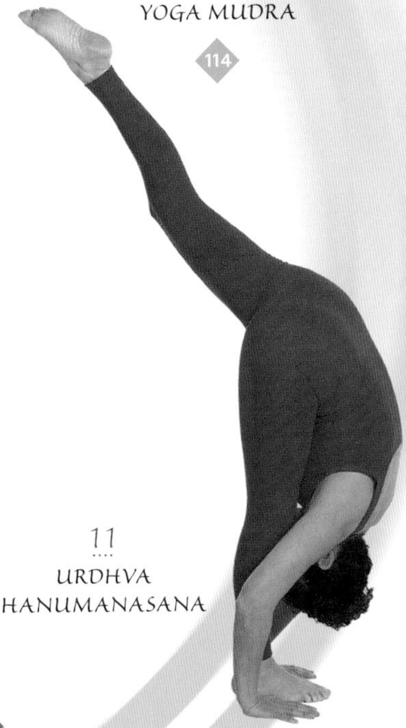

11
URDHVA
HANUMANASANA

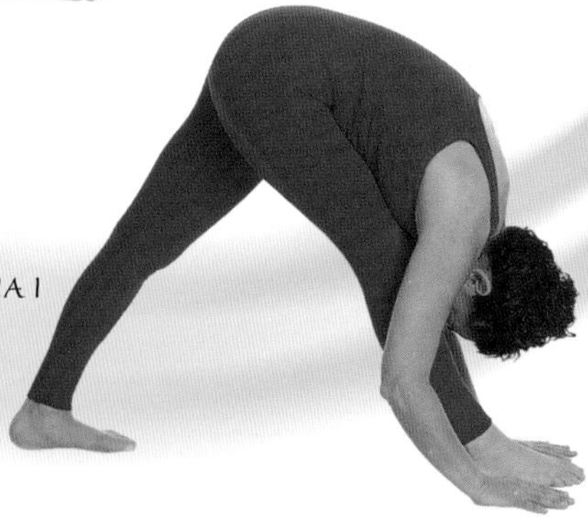

10
PARSVOTTANASANA I

◆ see FOCUS ON FLOWS section

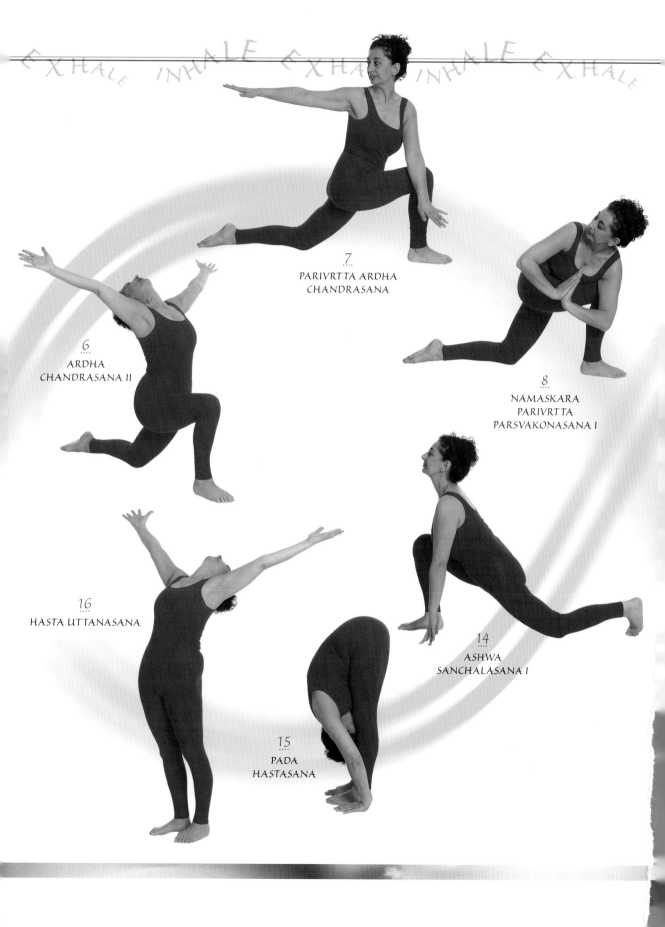

7.
PARIVRTTA ARDHA
CHANDRASANA

6
ARDHA
CHANDRASANA II

8.
NAMASKARA
PARIVRTTA
PARSVAKONASANA I

16
HASTA UTTANASANA

14
ASHWA
SANCHALASANA I

15
PADA
HASTASANA

INHALE EXHALE INHALE

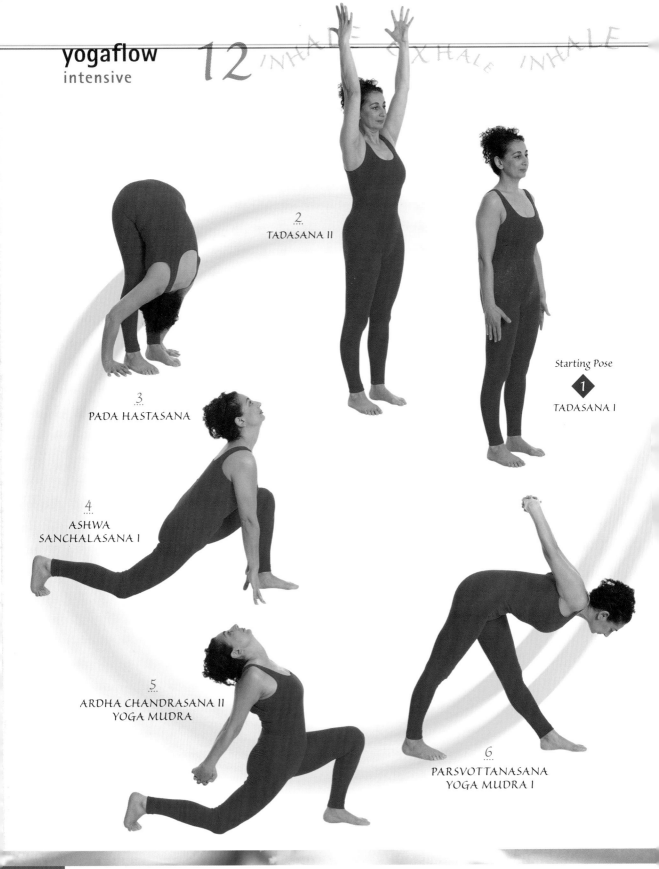

2.
TADASANA II

Starting Pose

1

TADASANA I

3.
PADA HASTASANA

4.
ASHWA
SANCHALASANA I

5.
ARDHA CHANDRASANA II
YOGA MUDRA

6.
PARSVOTTANASANA
YOGA MUDRA I

1 Inhale. Exhaling, start in TADASANA I (Mountain I).

2 Inhale. Exhaling, raise your arms in TADASANA II (Mountain II).

3 Inhale. Exhaling, fold your body forward in PADA HASTASANA (Standing Hand-to-Foot Forward Fold).

4 Inhale. Exhaling, step your right leg back in ASHWA SANCHALASANA I (Rider's I Lunge).

5 Inhale. Exhaling, interlock your hands behind your back. Move into ARDHA CHANDRASANA II YOGA MUDRA (Half-Moon II Seal of Yoga).

6 Inhale. Exhaling, straighten both legs, bringing your back foot in, in PARSVOTTANASANA YOGA MUDRA I (Pyramid Seal of Yoga I).

7 Inhale. Exhaling, move into PARSVOTTANASANA YOGA MUDRA II (Pyramid Seal of Yoga II).

8 Inhale. Exhaling, bend your left knee to a right angle. Bring your chest to your thighs and begin to lift your right leg. Inhale. Exhaling, straighten your left leg in URDHVA HANUMANASANA YOGA MUDRA (Upward-Standing Splits Seal of Yoga).

9 Repeat (7), then (6). Exhaling, release your right leg. Bring both hands down, pressing into your right toes, and move into ARDHA PARSVOTTANASANA (Half-Pyramid).

10 Inhale. Exhaling, move forward into ASHWA SANCHALASANA II (Rider's II High Lunge).

11 Inhale. Exhaling, step your right leg back into ADHO MUKHA SVANASANA (Downward-Facing Dog).

12 Inhaling, look up. Exhaling, step or jump forward, crossing your legs into SUKHASANA (Easy).

13 Inhale. Exhaling, extend both legs out in PASCHIMOTTANASANA (Seated Forward Fold).

14 Inhale. Exhaling, hold your big toes in each hand, bending your knees. Inhale. Exhaling, extend your legs upward, balancing on your tailbone, so that your body is V-shaped, in UBBAYA PADANGUSTHASANA (Raised Big Toes).

15 Inhale. Exhaling, with your toes still hooked, roll backward, extending your legs beyond your head. Inhale. Release your toe grip. Exhaling, move your arms behind your back, interlacing your fingers in HALASANA (Plough).

16 Inhale. Exhaling, lower your knees down by your ears. Keep your arms on your thighs, or move your lower arms over the back of your thighs, threading your hands through to cover your ears to listen to the sound of your breath in KARNAPIDASANA (Ear Pressure).

17 Inhale. Exhaling, leave this pose by lowering your legs with knees bent down to the ground. Inhale. Exhaling, move your arms under your buttocks, palms flat. Press your buttocks into your forearms and your forearms into the ground, lifting chest and head and placing the back of your head on the ground in MATSYASANA (Fish).

18 Inhale. Exhaling, release this pose, bending your knees up to your chest with your legs crossed. Inhaling, take your right foot into your left hand and your left foot into your right hand. Exhaling, sit up, rolling up onto your knees, palms flat, fingers on the ground. Bring your shins to rest on the backs of your upper arms, lifting your feet off the ground in KAKASANA (Crow). Look ahead.

19 Inhale. Exhaling, come into Majariasana (Table) and then SALAMBA KAKASANA (Inverted Crow).

20 Inhale. Exhaling, rest in GHARBHASANA (Child). Repeat the whole yogaflow sequence on your other side.

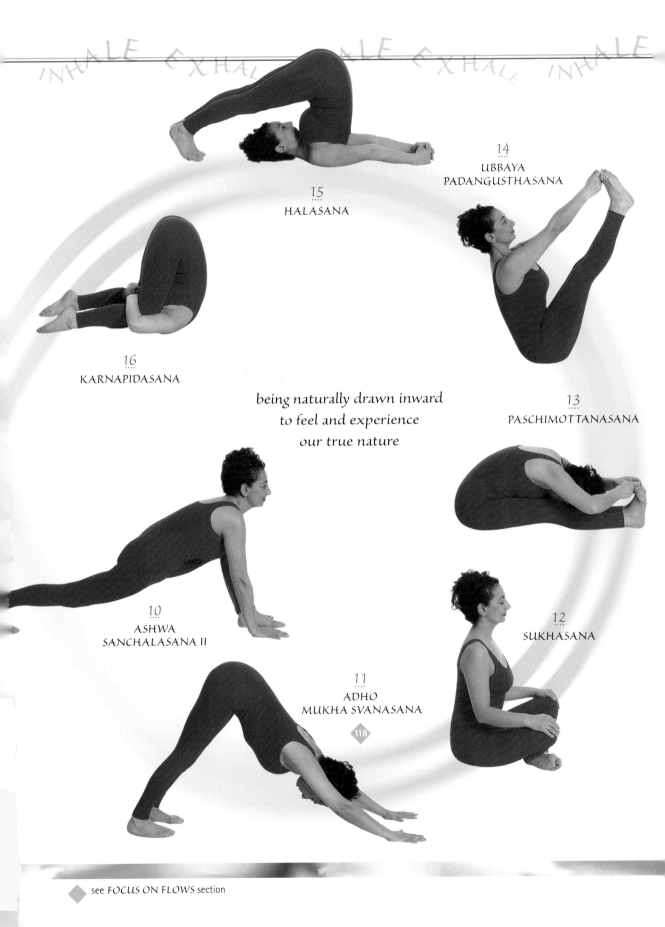

15
HALASANA

14
UBBAYA
PADANGUSTHASANA

16
KARNAPIDASANA

being naturally drawn inward
to feel and experience
our true nature

13
PASCHIMOTTANASANA

12
SUKHASANA

10
ASHWA
SANCHALASANA II

11
ADHO
MUKHA SVANASANA

118

◆ see FOCUS ON FLOWS section

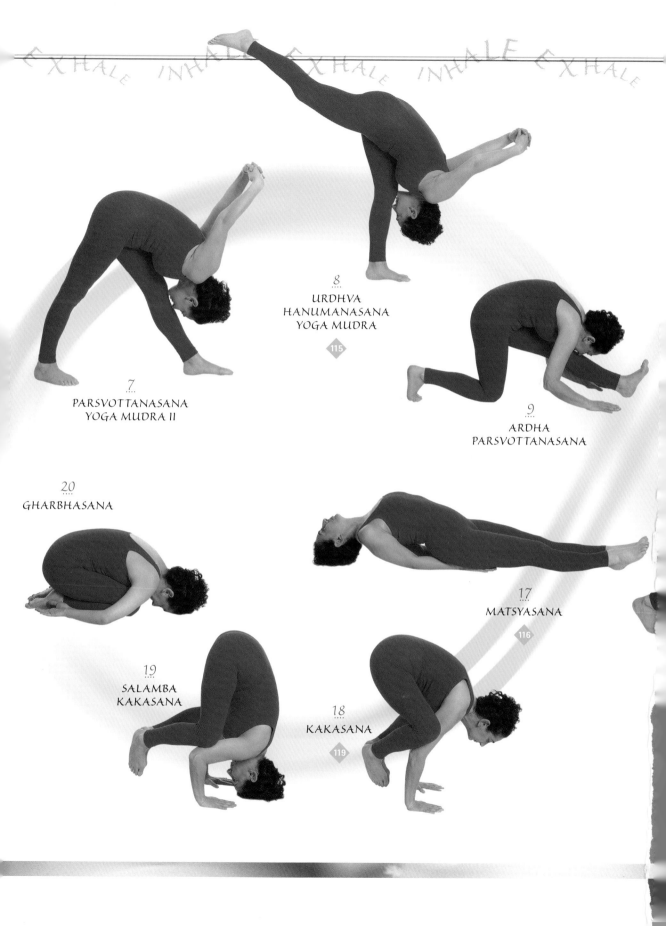

8.
URDHVA
HANUMANASANA
YOGA MUDRA
115

7.
PARSVOTTANASANA
YOGA MUDRA II

9.
ARDHA
PARSVOTTANASANA

20.
GHARBHASANA

17.
MATSYASANA
116

19.
SALAMBA
KAKASANA

18.
KAKASANA
119

fluidity in yogaflows

Once you are familiar with the sequences you can practice becoming more fluid in the yogaflows. This method involves the use of counting while breathing and moving. Establishing a comfortable count on both the inhale and the exhale, while moving into, holding and moving out of a pose, can have many benefits.

Creating fluidity

It is often the case, especially if a pose is challenging or strenuous, that your breath may be inhaled in one initial gulp and retained unconsciously while you adjust or move into a pose, then expelled all at once on the exhale when you release that pose. Unconsciously suspending your breath the whole time you are moving into your next pose can strain your lungs. The concept of fluidity, however, encourages more efficient, moment-by-moment breath management. A subtle awareness of the energy flow through your body creates a connection between your mind, which is focused on the practice, and your body and breath, which are flowing together synergistically. Breathing becomes seamless and circular, with little space between the inhale and the exhale. Awareness increases on all levels. In middle breathing, as the breath comes into your trachea, the action of pairs of intercostal muscles, used for inhalation and exhalation respectively, encourages your ribcage to move outward, downward and laterally as air is taken into your lungs. Your sternum lifts and moves forward as your diaphragm contracts or flattens. Your abdomen is only slightly distended as air enters your lungs, pressing your abdominal organs downward into your abdominal cavity.

Make full use of your breathing apparatus—thorax, lungs, ribs, intercostal and abdominal muscles, sternum and diaphragm—during middle breathing. Too deep a breath bypasses your thorax and fully distends your abdomen as air is taken down into your lower lungs. Too shallow a breath uses only the top half of your chest.

Initially, a steady count of four might be optimal on both the inhale and the exhale. This can be gradually increased to suit longer breathing rhythms, but an equal ratio of inhalation to exhalation is recommended. As in music, when learning rhythm, external counting and tapping are readily encouraged but are later discarded once rhythm has been internalized. The same applies to fluidity.

Find a type of breathing—seamless, rhythmic and effortless—which you find it easy to work and move with. Because breathing is always present, it is important to establish this constancy.

Using fluidity

Stage I Dynamic (Moving) Travel in or out of your pose with the inhale or the exhale, accordingly counting with your optimum number. Continue in this way during the whole yogaflow sequence.

Stage II Dynamic (Holding) As above, except hold your pose for a comfortable number of breaths, counting all the while, until your count has become internalized. Travel out of your pose with the inhale or the exhale, accordingly counting with your optimum number. Continue in this way during the whole yogaflow sequence.

MAHAT YOGA PRANAYAMA
three-part breath, stage II

The three-part breath cycle consolidates full yogic breath by breaking it down into its different components. Regular practice increases lung capacity.

body poses   These help isolate those body areas where your breath can be felt.

hand mudras   Also known as psycho-neural finger locks, these hand movements have been used across cultures throughout antiquity: in healing practices, dances, prayers, religious ceremonies, rituals and in communication. Fingers contain thousands of nerve endings which transmit energy, hence their extensive use in the art of healing. When connected, they unite various nerve channels in the sympathetic and parasympathetic nervous systems. A circuit of energy is produced, re-directed from your hands to your brain and back again. *Mudras* control different lobular sections of your lungs. The respiratory center in your brain, located at the medulla oblongata (brain stem), is divided into three areas—lower, middle and upper—controlling your abdominal, intercostal (diaphragmatic) and apical (clavicular) breathing respectively *(see pages 90–91)*. These areas can awaken the most dormant and unused parts of the "primitive" brain around your brain stem, stimulating access to unconscious and conditioned reflexes.

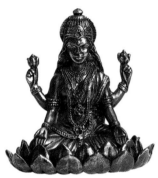

One of the most sought-after deities in Hindu mythology, Lakshmi is the goddess of wealth, fortune, royal power and beauty. She is invoked to bring fame and prosperity and is generous in bestowing abundance and bounty.

Apart from re-channelling energy from within, *mudras* work to remove instinctive habits which impede internal growth and to enhance a deeper state of relaxation and general awareness. This process redresses the balance of subtle energies, encouraging a deeper meditative state.

Different sounds are associated with each *mudra* and section of your lungs *(see pages 90–91)*. The sounds produced increase in strength, vigor and weight as breathing becomes prolonged and deeper, coming in fully after each sound on the exhale.

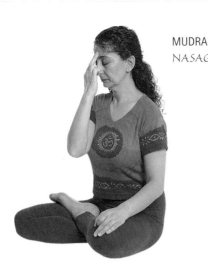

MUDRA
NASAGRA & GYAN

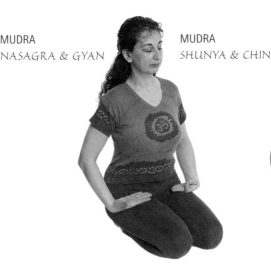

MUDRA
SHUNYA & CHIN

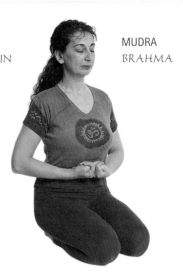

MUDRA
BRAHMA

How to begin

Refer to the chart *(see pages 90–91)* on yoga *mudras* and *asanas*. Practice the *asanas* and integrate them into your daily routine. Feel the corresponding parts of your lung being activated as you hold each pose (poses 1–3). *Mudras*, together with their corresponding sounds, promote a calmer body and mind. Practice them after *asana* but before *pranayama*. Sit in *Sukhasana* (Easy) or *Vajrasana* (Thunderbolt) and assume the *mudras* in sequential order.

To gain an awareness of the energy center for a particular area, begin with a few rounds of natural breath and move to a conscious, deliberate breath for 3–5 rounds. Add the corresponding sound for each *mudra*, preserving volume and intensity levels to the end of your breath. Allow it to fade off naturally. Repeat for 3–5 rounds. Practice *Shunya* (Void or Empty) *Mudra* at the start of the *mudra* sequence or at the end, after the sounds. Use only one open palm, with the other in *Gyan Mudra* (Seal of Knowledge).

Ensure fingers are strong, with palms resting upwards on your knees or thighs. For *Brahma Mudra*, knuckles should touch with your hands held up against your body, above your navel.

deepening your breath cycle

This overview looks at the impact of physical, neurological and energetic aspects of using hand mudras. Practice each body pose to identify individual stages with the corresponding lung section activated. Continue by introducing mudras and sounds for an overall effect.

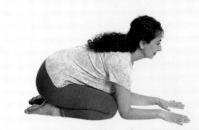

asanas (body poses)	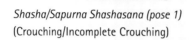	
	Shasha/Sapurna Shashasana (pose 1) (Crouching/Incomplete Crouching)	*Purna Shashasana (pose 2)* (Extended Crouching)
lung section	Lower	Middle
hand mudras (seals)	Chin	Chin Maya
sound/energy center	Aah/Root/Sacral/Sexual	Ooh/Heart/Lungs
brain section	Autonomic nerves	Cerebral cortex
impulse arising from	Phrenic nerve (the cervical nerve which enters the thorax and passes into the diaphragm); the motor nerve to the diaphragm; the sensory fibers to the pericardium	Vagus or pneumastric nerve (tenth cranial); mixed nerve (motor and sensory)
brain location	Lower brain (diaphragmatic breathing)	Middle brain (intercostal/diaphragmatic breathing)

Practice poses 1 and 2. Keep your chin parallel to the ground. In these poses, your head presses the respiratory center in your medulla oblongata.

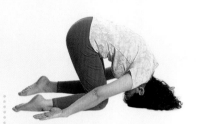

Pari-Purna Shashasana (pose 3) (Complete Extended Crouching)

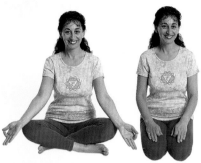

Sukhasana (Easy) *(pose 4)* or *Vajrasana* (Thunderbolt) *(pose 5)*

Upper	Three parts	One lung
Adhi	Brahma	Shunya
Hmm/Head/Throat	Ahoomm/Aum/Crown	No sound
Cerebral cortex	Medulla oblongata	Medulla oblongata
Conscious brain, mental impulses, gray matter.	Creative impulses of the brain and the central nervous system.	
Upper brain (apical/clavicular breathing)	Whole brain The three sections combine into a complete breath (lower, middle and upper sections inflate consecutively).	Individually emphasizes the subtle action of each lung.

NADI SHODHANA PRANAYAMA
nostril breath

During this energy-cleansing practice, also known as "silent *pranayama*", your breath becomes inaudible or silent.

How to begin
Single nostril breath with Nasagra (Nose Tip) Mudra (see page 89)

Sitting in a comfortable, cross-legged position, place your left hand on your knee in *Gyan Mudra* (Seal of Knowledge). With your right hand, using either *Nasagra Mudra* or *Gyan Mudra*, close your right nostril with your thumb. Breathe in and out through your left nostril for 5 rounds (one round equals one inhale and one exhale). Close your left nostril with your ring finger and little finger and open your right nostril. Breathe in and out through your right nostril for 5 rounds. Equalize the in- and out-breaths by counting as you breathe in and out. Release the *mudra* and breathe for 5 rounds through both nostrils. Repeat for 5 rounds.

Alternate nostril breath

Sitting in a comfortable, cross-legged position, place your left hand on your knee in *Gyan Mudra* (Seal of Knowledge). Close your right nostril and open your left nostril. Inhale through your left nostril and close it. Open your right nostril, exhaling through it. Inhale through your right nostril and close it. Open your left nostril, exhaling through it. This equals one round. Equalize the in- and out-breaths by counting as you breathe in and out. Repeat for up to 10 rounds, increasing over time to 10 minutes twice daily.

Benefits
Nostril breath encourages inner calm by lengthening the breath; provides a good preparation for meditation; detoxifies the blood; increases the supply of oxygen to all the body's systems; optimizes brain functioning by purifying the cerebral cells.

KAPALABHATHI PRANAYAMA
shining skull breath

This practice is a *kriya* (cleansing action) and a *pranayama* (breath control), bringing oxygen to the frontal parts of your brain.

How to begin

From a comfortable, seated or kneeling position, place your hand on your abdomen. Feel the natural movement of your breath. Exhale forcefully through your nostrils and not your mouth.

Contract your abdominal muscles toward your spine, expelling all air through both nostrils. Your diaphragm moves upward, contracting to release all air from your lungs. Observe the natural rebound action of these muscles on the inhale as your diaphragm flattens to let air rush in during passive inhalation. Repeat for up to 10 rounds. As your practice develops, increase the pace and bring the number of expulsions to 15. Practice for several rounds (one round consists of 10–15 expulsions plus three normal deep breaths in and out). Repeat for up to 5 rounds.

Benefits

Shining skull breath cleanses the sinuses, throat and nasal passages; improves circulation and detoxifies the blood; benefits the nervous system; relieves sleepiness; encourages a clearer, calmer and more focused mind. The diaphragmatic movement on the exhale massages heart and lungs. The impact of the active exhalation on abdominal muscles tones and massages all digestive organs.

Notes

This practice is not recommended for those with high blood pressure, heart disease, epilepsy, stomach ulcers, hernias, stroke patients, or pregnant or menstruating women.

relaxation 1 *earth*

The body is said to be the "temple of the Divine or the Spirit".
By looking after it, you nurture its "sacred spark", that inner light
which reflects through your whole being. If you neglect it, it
begins to fade.

Meditation and yoga practice guide us toward an inner reflective
state—a safe place or sanctuary. The earth is also a temple and holds
all living beings within it. By attuning to the earth and her dynamics
you learn to observe how, as a living organism, you too, resonate
with the earth.

the entry Entering the sanctuary of the earth is no different to entering the
sanctuary of the body. Find a space outdoors to feel the benefits of
this relaxation at a deeper level. Feel the earth, her pulse, her living
energy, and all the surrounding elements. Find a secluded spot and
settle down in *Savasana* (Corpse) or *Sukhasana* (Easy) and let go.

taking root Allow yourself to open like the petals of a flower ready to receive
the pulse of the earth. Connect fully with the moment to feel at one
with nature.

> *May I be solid as the rock*
> *May I be strong as the tree*
> *May I be light as the air*
> *May I sustain myself as the earth sustains herself*
> *May I develop an acute sense of hearing*
> *May I develop a clarity of vision*
> *Then may I attune to a deeper inner seeing and hearing*
> *Sinking into safety, gaining support, sustainability from the earth*
> *Opening to lightness, clarity, abundance from all around me*
> *Receiving an all-encompassing generosity from All That Is.*

the return Come back to an awareness of your body lying on the ground.
Begin to deepen your breath so it becomes active. Move your fingers
and toes slowly, bringing your knees to your chest, rocking from
side-to-side. Release the pose when ready.

relaxation 2 *ground and space*

This practice helps you move beyond the limitations of your physical body. It widens your perspective and awareness in all directions and promotes an all-encompassing connection with the earth and with yourself.

grounding Settle in *Savasana* (Corpse). Let your breath become natural and spontaneous. Travel through your body, finding your grounding points (those parts of your body which touch the ground): your heels, calves, thighs, buttocks; parts of your back; your shoulders; the backs of your arms; the backs of your hands; the back of your head. Travel back and forth between them and ground yourself through these points. Stay momentarily grounded at each point, "deepening" and "rooting" each part into the ground at a time.

space Concentrate on the space in and around your body, starting with your feet. See and feel the space between these body parts and the ground: your ankles; the back of your knees; the small of your back; the backs of your wrists; your neck. Feel and see the space between these body parts: your toes; your legs; your arms and the sides of your body; your fingers; your ears and shoulders; your chin and throat. Feel and see the space in your palms; your ears; your nostrils; your mouth; around your eyes; and finally, the space all around your body. Repeat as in the grounding above. Return to each body part individually and hold. Begin to open and expand the space all around you. Widen these space points.

the union Recall your grounding and space points. Visualize deepening the former and expanding the latter. See how this feels. Feel the union of your grounding points, which have merged with the earth, and your space points, which have merged with the space around you. Feel cocooned, nourished, held between the two. Rest here a while.

the return Come back to an awareness of your body and your breath, paying attention to your nostrils as your breath deepens. Initiate small movements in your joints when you feel ready. Return safely.

meditation 1 *being*

The great Indian sage Patanjali, responsible for systematizing the practice of yoga, defined meditation as *"Yoga chitta vritti nirodah".* This translates into several meanings: yoga is the stilling of the mind, yoga is peace of mind, and meditation is an unbroken stream of awareness or consciousness.

settling Sit in a comfortable position with your buttocks supported on a block (or cushion) to raise your hips and align your back. Settle in.

alignment and Ground yourself through those body points resting on the ground.
grounding Take root through the earth as a tree puts down roots. Draw energy from the earth like sap rising up through a tree trunk. Allow this energy to travel up through your spine, your trunk, into your head. Imagine an opening on the top of your head, energy pushing up and through it, opening outward like the canopy of a tree. Feel connected with the earth and the sky.

stillness Find a space of inner tranquility where you can "dock" like a boat in search of somewhere to moor. Turn your engine off. From here, observe your mental chattering and allow it to rise, until it quietens.

breath Come into an awareness of your breath. Observe this continuous, life-giving force. Float your attention on the ebb and flow of your breath as it irons out any creases in your mind, body or spirit. Let go and connect with the "here and now".

here and now Focus on the "here and now". Feel the energy within you. Find and identify a place inside of you which captures the present moment.

the experience Grounded in the present moment, note any insights, new perspectives, intuitive knowledge that comes your way. To return, bring your awareness back to your breath and your body. Release.

meditation 2 *finding the gap*

Sit in a comfortable, seated position. Settle your body, align and ground it. Come into an awareness of your natural breath. Begin watching the inhale and the exhale: how they rise and fall, spontaneously, effortlessly. Take your time. After the inhale, notice the small gap until the exhale occurs. After the exhale, there is also a small gap before the inhale reoccurs. Try to find these gaps. Allow this to happen spontaneously without forcing it. This is why the use of natural breath is emphasized here.

the gap Once you have found the gap, stay with it, feel it. If your mind wanders, come back to your breath. Find that space again and focus on it. Where does it come from? Does it have a shape which you can see? Does it reflect a feeling that you can experience? Stay there. Let your attention move from the inhale to the gap, and from the exhale to the gap. When you are in that space, observe your breath. The inhale and the exhale occur around it. Widen it. Observe what happens to your awareness and your consciousness. Shift your awareness away from your breath to the gap. You know you are breathing, you can feel it. See it happening spontaneously as your awareness is focused on the gap, the space.

> *Coming to the place*
> *Where all things arise*
> *Where all things return*
> *Find the moment now, find the gap*
> *Observe when you have lost the moment, lost the gap*
> *Find the moment, find the gap—again and again and again*
> *Until the gap is you, and you are it.*

the return Bring your attention back to your body and your breath, drawing attention to what surrounds you. Become aware of nearby sounds, smells and tastes. Begin to deepen your breath and, when you are ready, release.

visualization 1 *name and form*

Take a comfortable seated or supine position. Get settled, aligned and grounded. Become aware of the breath. Open up to what you are experiencing right now. Watch how your body becomes still and your mind introspective and quiet. Stay in this space for a while, savoring the feeling of your body and the quietness of your mind. Become fully aware of yourself from a physical point of view. Fully embrace this body that you call "yours". Become aware of the name you go by, your marital status, your family, your profession, your hobbies, your house, your possessions, your children, your pets: everything that is associated with your name and form. Discover the package that defines "you".

forget who you are Temporarily suspend all mental images and stories that lead you back to your name and form. Willingly try this. What picture appears before you in your mind's eye as you remove your "coat" of name and form? Where do you "dock", where have you arrived? What is there? What new experience of self do you see and feel standing naked before yourself? Observe. As your mind constantly pulls you back to name and form and all manner of social restrictions, keep letting go, returning back to the space where you docked, to that energy, that special place. Once you are there, feel it.

tune into your essence Be aware that you are feeling that essence and that light: the quiet, still place where all is well, where there is equanimity, tranquility and love. See that in this place both everything and nothing are contained. Are you able to come into a clearer picture of who you really are? Can you redefine yourself in view of the experiences observed at the dropping of name and form?

the return Slowly bring your attention back to your body and the breath at your nostrils. Breathe in, moving slowly to come out of the process. Realize how you feel, experience and savor it.

visualization 2 *seat of life*

Sit or lie comfortably with your body settled and aligned.

imagine the chair   This is the chair of your life. Picture its color, texture and design.

sitting on the chair   This is your life. Do you feel supported or not? Feel the chair, below and around you. Feel your life. See your life. How has it been so far? Let events flood into your awareness. Try to observe them naturally rather than trying to relive them. Notice any feelings, people or situations which arise with detachment. Become an observer, a "witness" to what you see.

something is beckoning   See a strong light beckoning you in the distance. Imagine you leave the chair. Notice any feelings of attachment or other feelings which may arise as you begin to move. Then journey towards the light, which gets stronger as you approach and dimmer as you veer off the path. Travel the path, making sure that you stay on it without getting sidetracked. Observe whatever is presented to you without becoming involved. Use your skills of detached observation to move through your journey to get to the light.

inside the light   Once you have arrived at the light, sit in it, feel its substance, experience its glow, merge with it. Stay here. Observe.

looking back to the chair   Try to see the chair as symbolic of your life: somewhere you place yourself, where you take stock, where you rest. What is the seat of your life? Stay open to whatever message is being transmitted to you.

returning from the light   Come back from the light toward your chair. Notice whether there is any resistance to leave the light. Take note of why this may be before returning. Move toward your chair, sit down on it. Feel it, experience it. Return to an awareness of your body and the breath.

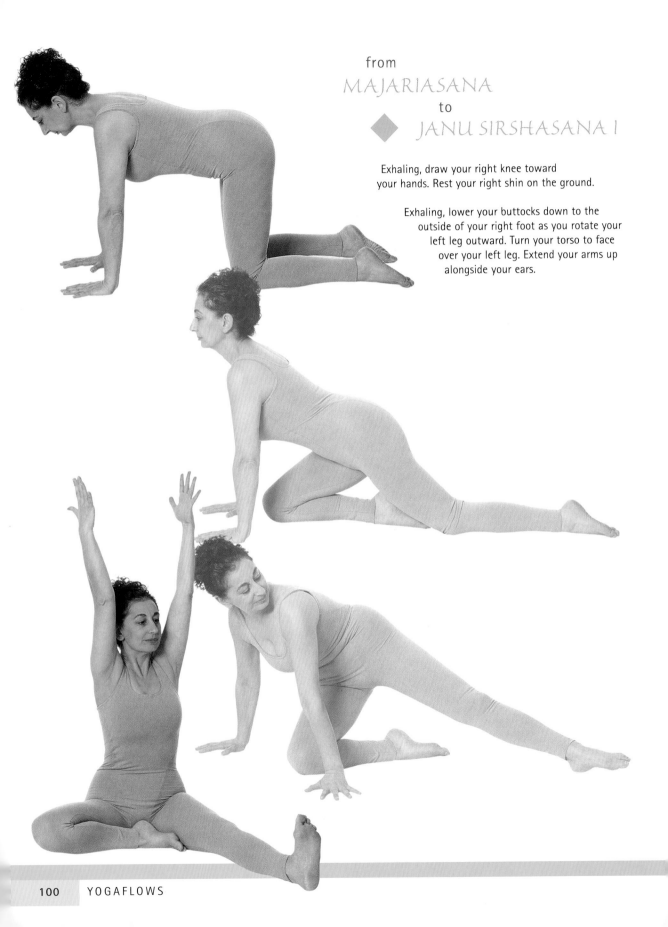

from
MAJARIASANA
to
◆ JANU SIRSHASANA I

Exhaling, draw your right knee toward
your hands. Rest your right shin on the ground.

Exhaling, lower your buttocks down to the
outside of your right foot as you rotate your
left leg outward. Turn your torso to face
over your left leg. Extend your arms up
alongside your ears.

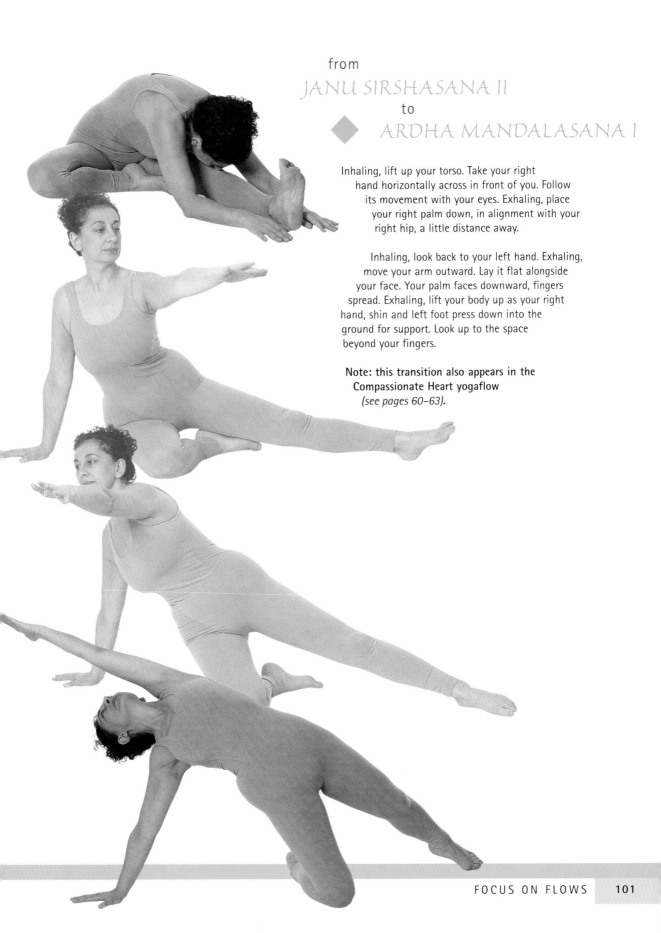

from
JANU SIRSHASANA II
to
◆ ARDHA MANDALASANA I

Inhaling, lift up your torso. Take your right hand horizontally across in front of you. Follow its movement with your eyes. Exhaling, place your right palm down, in alignment with your right hip, a little distance away.

Inhaling, look back to your left hand. Exhaling, move your arm outward. Lay it flat alongside your face. Your palm faces downward, fingers spread. Exhaling, lift your body up as your right hand, shin and left foot press down into the ground for support. Look up to the space beyond your fingers.

Note: this transition also appears in the Compassionate Heart yogaflow *(see pages 60–63).*

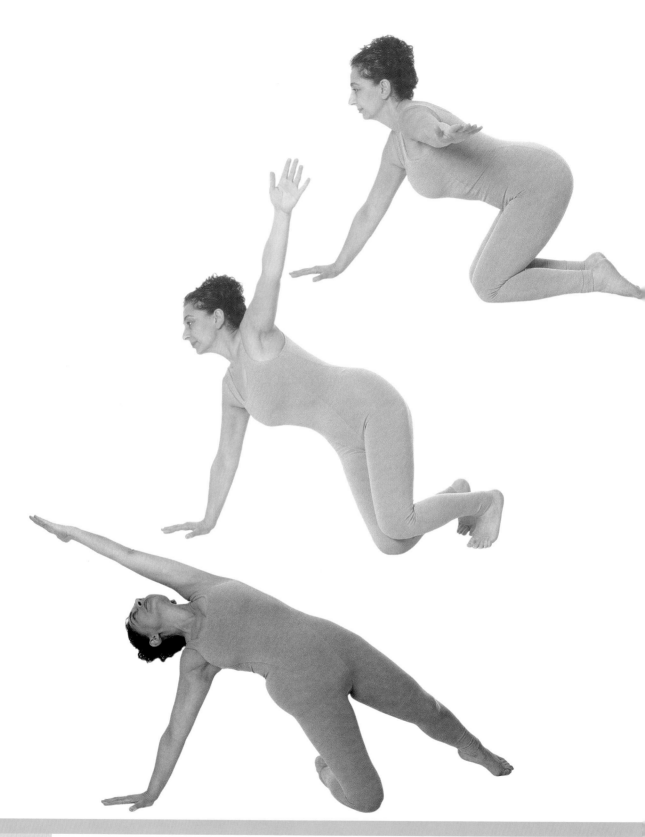

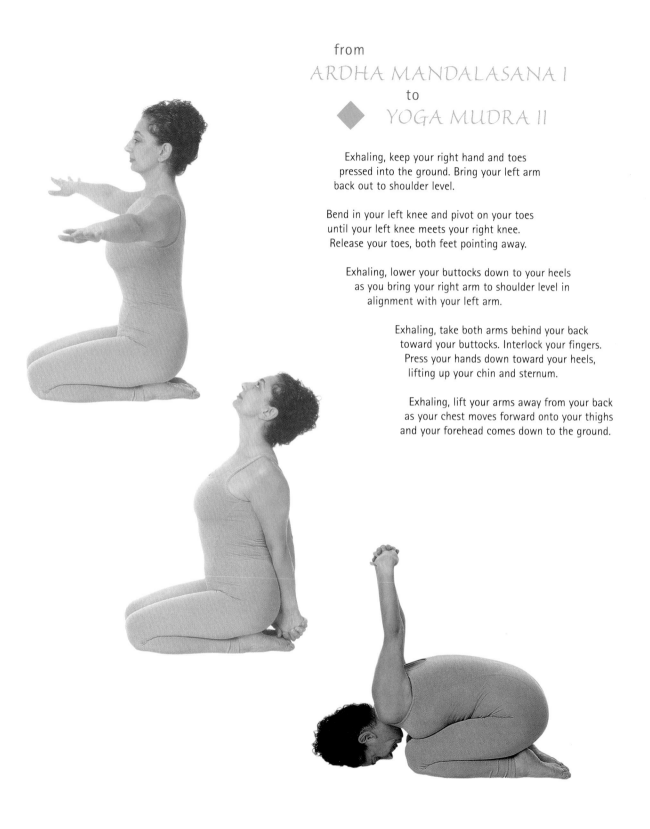

from
ARDHA MANDALASANA I
to
◆ YOGA MUDRA II

Exhaling, keep your right hand and toes pressed into the ground. Bring your left arm back out to shoulder level.

Bend in your left knee and pivot on your toes until your left knee meets your right knee. Release your toes, both feet pointing away.

Exhaling, lower your buttocks down to your heels as you bring your right arm to shoulder level in alignment with your left arm.

Exhaling, take both arms behind your back toward your buttocks. Interlock your fingers. Press your hands down toward your heels, lifting up your chin and sternum.

Exhaling, lift your arms away from your back as your chest moves forward onto your thighs and your forehead comes down to the ground.

from

PRASARITA PADOTTANASANA
to
◆ ASHWA SANCHALASANA II

Exhaling, turn your feet to the right by half-a-turn as you walk your hands around and bring your torso to rest on your right thigh.

Exhaling, place your hands either side of your right leg which is bent at a right angle. Look ahead.

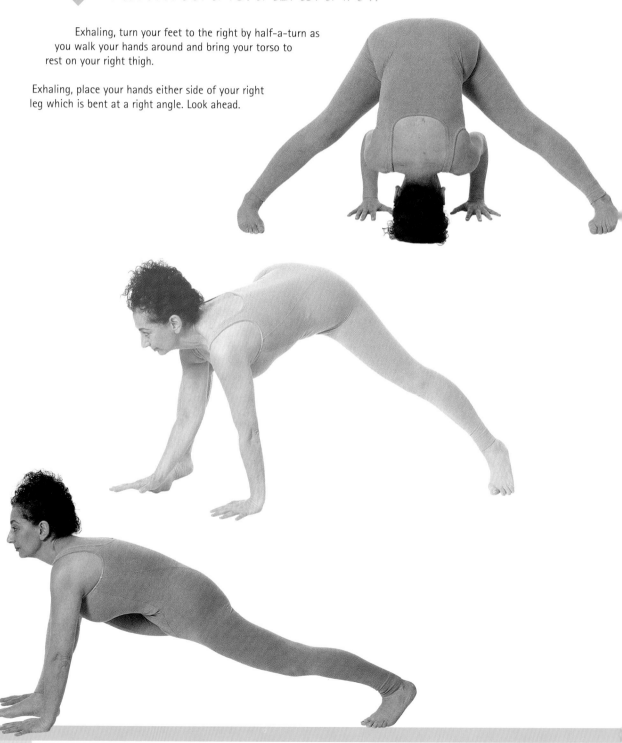

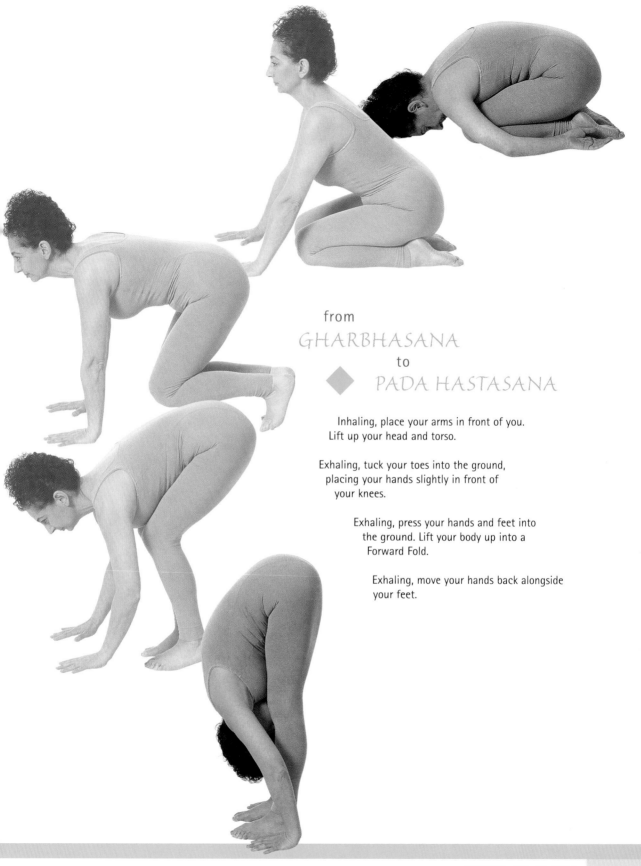

from
GHARBHASANA
to
◆ PADA HASTASANA

Inhaling, place your arms in front of you.
Lift up your head and torso.

Exhaling, tuck your toes into the ground,
placing your hands slightly in front of
your knees.

Exhaling, press your hands and feet into
the ground. Lift your body up into a
Forward Fold.

Exhaling, move your hands back alongside
your feet.

from
PADA HASTASANA
to
◆ NATARAJASANA I

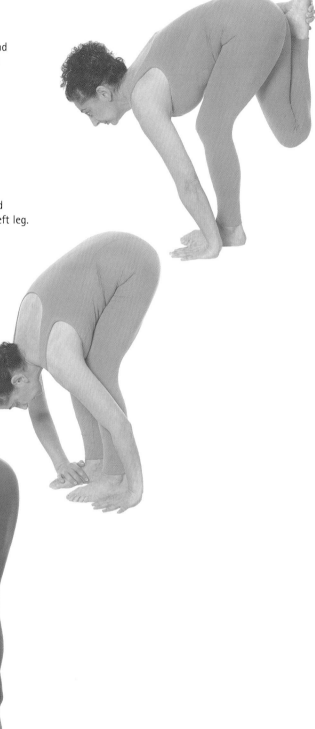

Inhaling, bend both knees, keeping your chest and thighs connected. Exhaling, place your right palm over your right foot, fingers facing to the left.

Exhaling, lift up your torso. Look ahead as your right heel is brought in toward your right buttock. Keep your left hand on the ground for balance.

Inhaling, keep your balance by focusing ahead of you. Slowly lift your left arm out in front.

Exhaling, begin to lift up your torso toward a horizontal position, straightening your left leg.

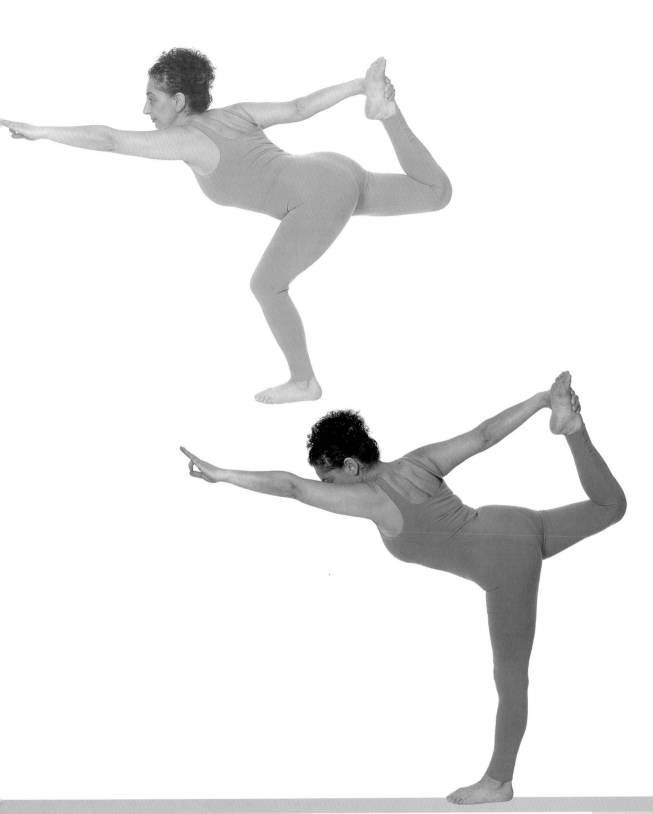

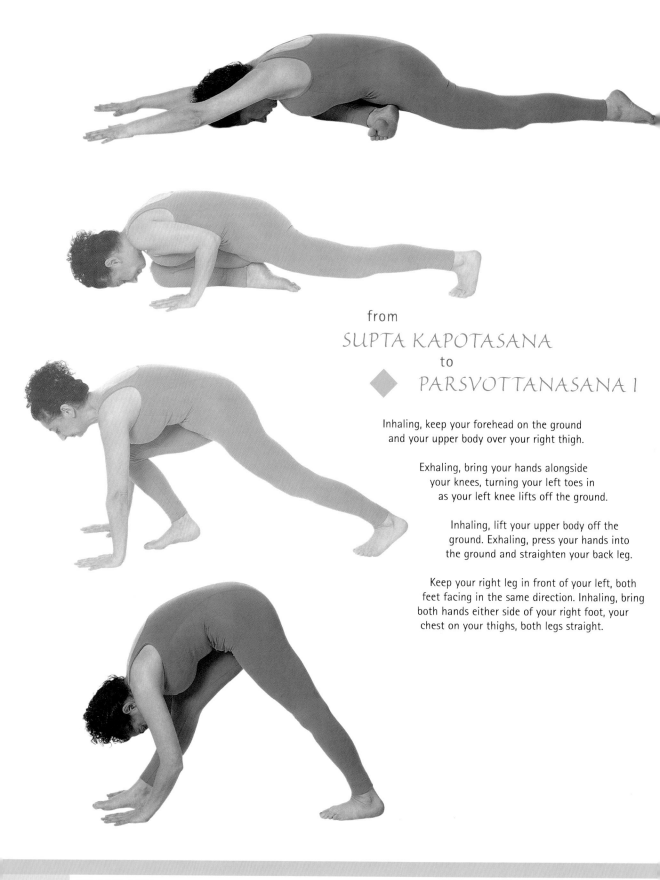

from
SUPTA KAPOTASANA
to
◆ PARSVOTTANASANA I

Inhaling, keep your forehead on the ground
and your upper body over your right thigh.

Exhaling, bring your hands alongside
your knees, turning your left toes in
as your left knee lifts off the ground.

Inhaling, lift your upper body off the
ground. Exhaling, press your hands into
the ground and straighten your back leg.

Keep your right leg in front of your left, both
feet facing in the same direction. Inhaling, bring
both hands either side of your right foot, your
chest on your thighs, both legs straight.

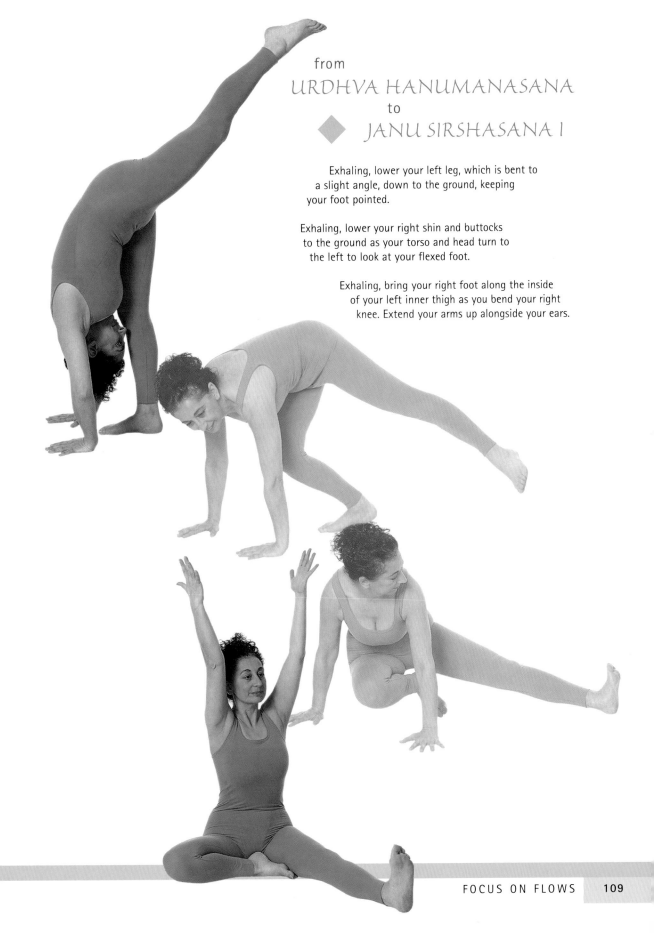

from
URDHVA HANUMANASANA
to
◆ JANU SIRSHASANA I

Exhaling, lower your left leg, which is bent to
a slight angle, down to the ground, keeping
your foot pointed.

Exhaling, lower your right shin and buttocks
to the ground as your torso and head turn to
the left to look at your flexed foot.

Exhaling, bring your right foot along the inside
of your left inner thigh as you bend your right
knee. Extend your arms up alongside your ears.

from
DHANURASANA
to
◆ GHARBHASANA

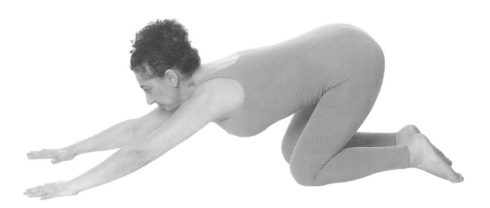

Release your hands and lower your legs down to the ground. Place your hands either side of your chest.

Exhaling, press your hands into the ground and lift your chest off the ground. Move your buttocks back toward your heels.

Place your arms alongside your body with your hands by your ankles and your forehead on the ground.

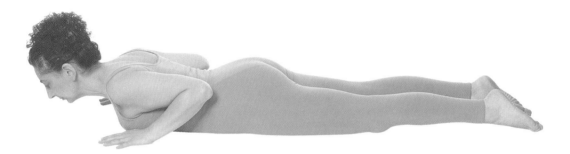

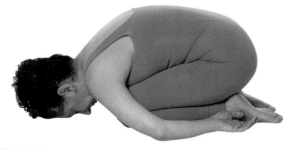

from
ARDHA MANDALASANA II
to
◆ ARDHA MATSYENDRASANA I

Exhaling, bring your left leg around to the front of your body.

Place your left foot on the outside of your right knee. As your foot touches the ground, move your right foot out to the left, creating a space behind your legs in which to lower your buttocks.

Exhaling, lower your buttocks to the ground, with your left leg crossed over your right leg. Allow your left hand to move behind your back. Place your palm on the ground, fingers facing away from your back. Extend your right arm upward.

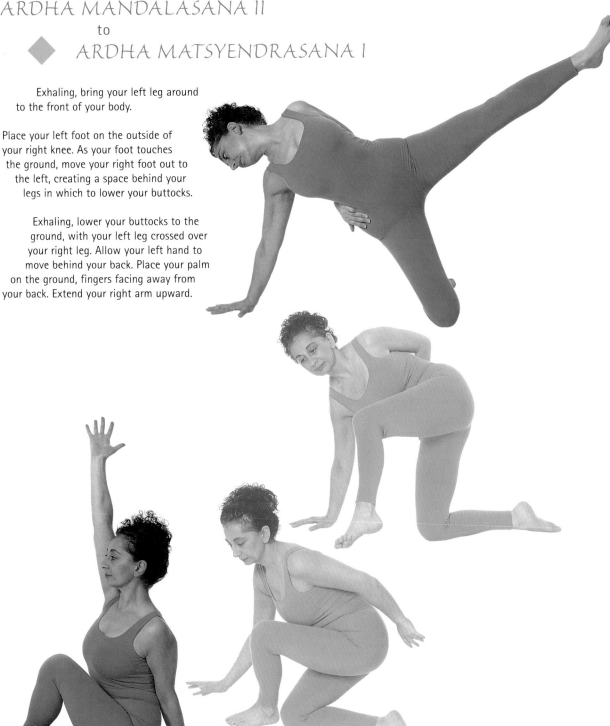

from
ARDHA MATSYENDRASANA II
to
 ## YOGA MUDRA I

Inhaling, release both your arms. Exhaling, rotate both arms around to the right, palms to the ground.

Lift up your buttocks and rotate your knees and body to the right by half-a-turn.

Bring your knees together, lowering your buttocks onto your heels. Inhaling, with your arms in front, prepare to sweep them behind your back toward the soles of your feet.

Exhaling, interlace your fingers, pressing your hands down toward your feet as you lift up your chin and sternum.

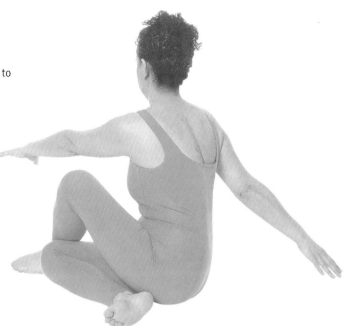

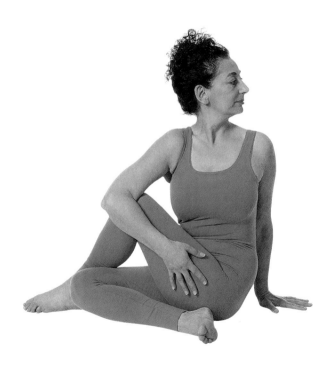

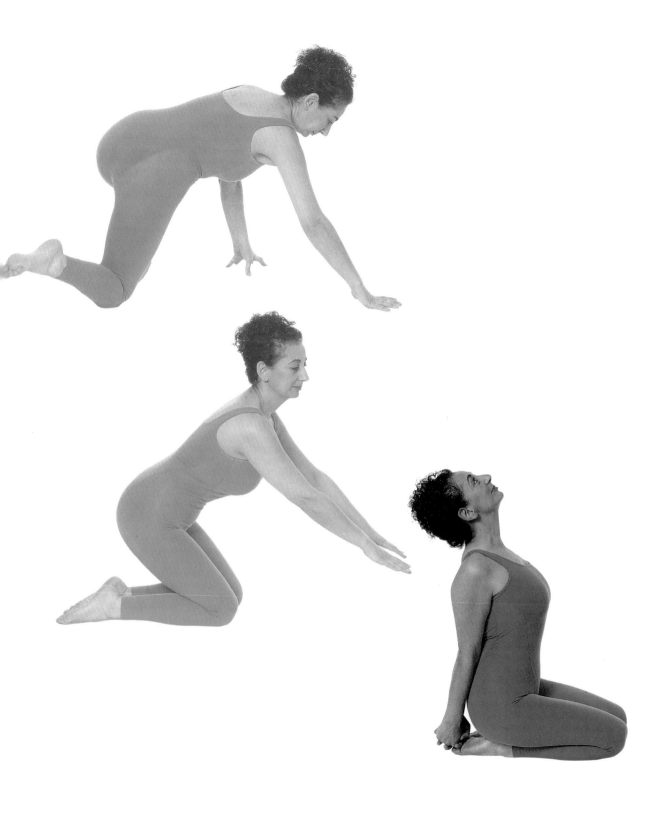

from

PRASARITA PADOTTANASANA YOGA MUDRA
to
◆ UTTHITA EKAPADA ANGUSTHASANA

Exhaling, release your arms, palms to the ground.
Exhaling, come up on tiptoes as your body rotates over
your right leg, knees bent, and your right arm moves to
the outside of your right leg, your fingers to the ground.

Exhaling, bring your left knee to the ground, sit back
toward your left heel, keeping your toes tucked.
Extend your right leg in front, keeping your torso
upright. Clasp your right foot with both hands,
raising it off the ground, as you take your
weight further back into your left foot,
flattening it on the ground.

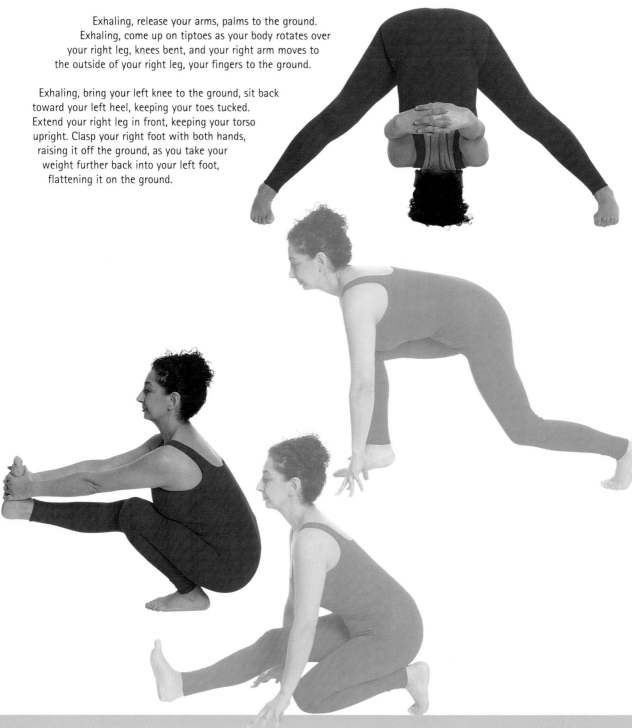

from
URDHVA HANUMANASANA YOGA MUDRA
to
ARDHA PARSVOTTANASANA

Exhaling, bring your right leg
down. Exhaling, release your
arms, placing your fingers or palms
on the ground, either side of your left
foot. Exhaling, bend both knees, placing your
right knee on the ground. Exhaling, tuck your
right toes into the ground. Lean your body weight
back toward your right heel.

Exhaling, extend your left leg out in front and
flex your foot. Place your hands alongside your
left leg. Exhaling, extend and fold forward.
Bring your arms out in front.

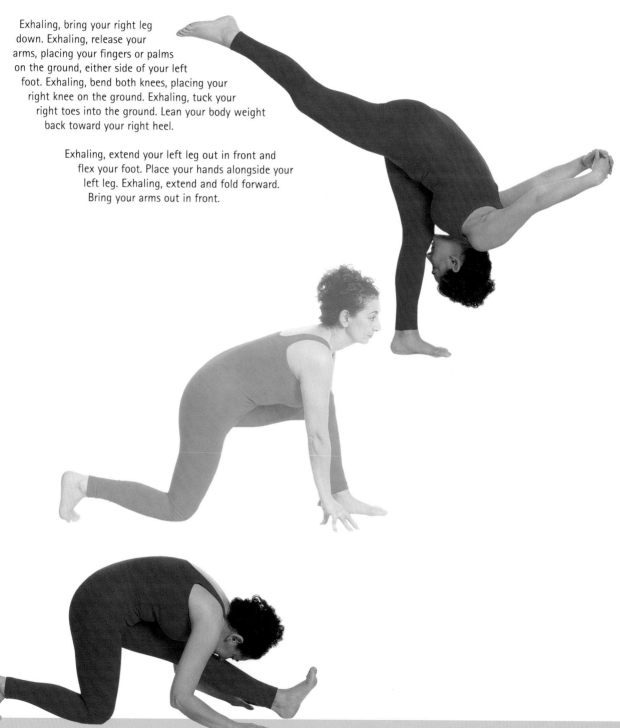

from
MATSYASANA
to
 KAKASANA

Exhaling, bring your head and torso down to
the ground. Release your arms from beneath your
body. Bring your arms out to the sides, palms up.

Exhaling, bring your knees toward your chest,
crossing your feet over your buttocks. Inhaling,
clasp the top of your right foot with your
left hand, the top of your left foot with your
right hand, palms down, elbows on the
outside of your body.

Exhaling, keep your head tucked into your
chest, then tightly pull your feet in toward
your buttocks and sit up, legs crossed, placing
both hands down in front of you.

Exhaling, uncross your legs. Come up on tiptoes.
Lift up your tailbone. Bend your arms. Lift your
feet off the floor as you balance your knees on the
backs of your upper arms.

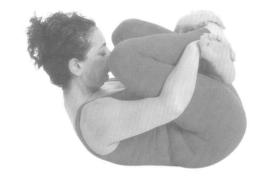

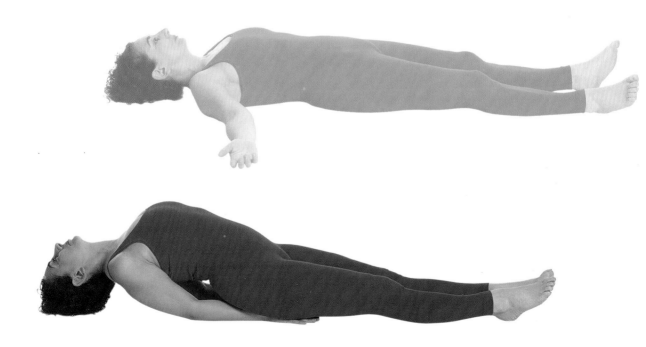

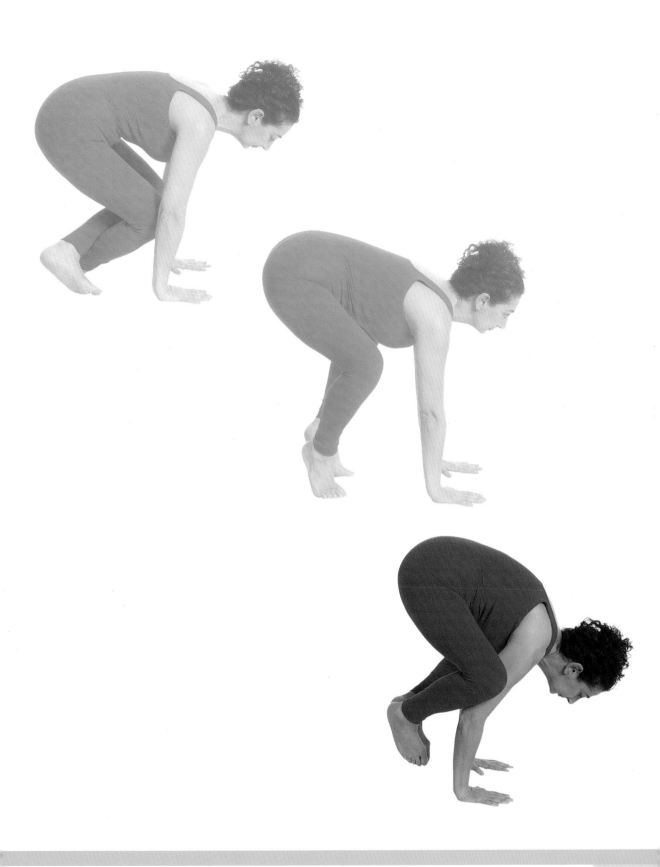

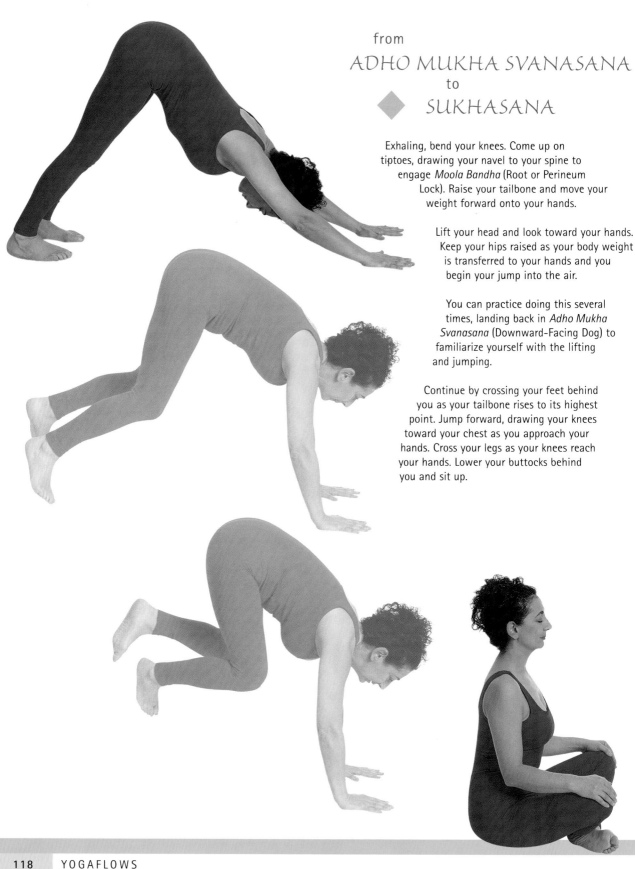

from
ADHO MUKHA SVANASANA
to
◆ SUKHASANA

Exhaling, bend your knees. Come up on tiptoes, drawing your navel to your spine to engage *Moola Bandha* (Root or Perineum Lock). Raise your tailbone and move your weight forward onto your hands.

Lift your head and look toward your hands. Keep your hips raised as your body weight is transferred to your hands and you begin your jump into the air.

You can practice doing this several times, landing back in *Adho Mukha Svanasana* (Downward-Facing Dog) to familiarize yourself with the lifting and jumping.

Continue by crossing your feet behind you as your tailbone rises to its highest point. Jump forward, drawing your knees toward your chest as you approach your hands. Cross your legs as your knees reach your hands. Lower your buttocks behind you and sit up.

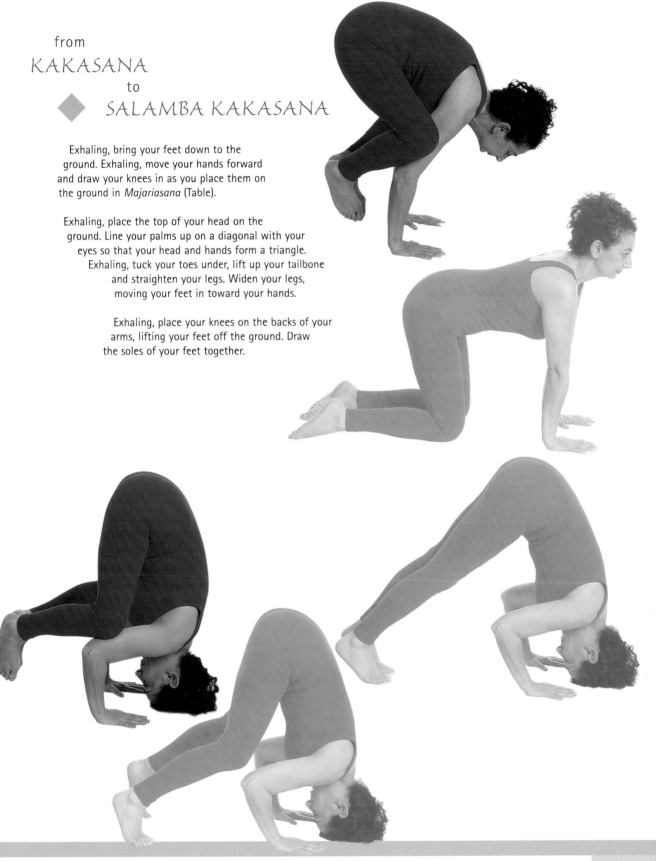

from
KAKASANA
to
◆ SALAMBA KAKASANA

Exhaling, bring your feet down to the ground. Exhaling, move your hands forward and draw your knees in as you place them on the ground in *Majariasana* (Table).

Exhaling, place the top of your head on the ground. Line your palms up on a diagonal with your eyes so that your head and hands form a triangle. Exhaling, tuck your toes under, lift up your tailbone and straighten your legs. Widen your legs, moving your feet in toward your hands.

Exhaling, place your knees on the backs of your arms, lifting your feet off the ground. Draw the soles of your feet together.

ASANAS 1-10
glossary of poses

1 ADHO MUKHA SVANASANA
Downward-Facing Dog

Keeping your legs and arms straight (hip- and shoulder-width apart respectively), feet and arms parallel, spread your toes and fingers. Lift up your tailbone, pelvis in Dog Tilt, as your chest moves between your arms toward your thighs. Lift your shoulders back, away from your ears, heels toward or on the ground.

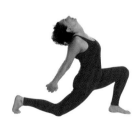

2 ADVASANA
Reversed Corpse

Assume a prostrate position with your forehead to the ground. Extend your arms out in front, parallel and shoulder-width apart, palms down, legs relaxed, feet flat.

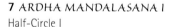

3 ARDHA CHANDRASANA I
Half-Moon I

Keeping your feet less than hip-width apart, stretch your arms up overhead, alongside your ears. Interlace your fingers. Extend your index fingers, cross your thumbs and press upward through your fingers. Keep your elbows straight and your shoulders down. Moving to the right, press your left foot into the ground as your left hip presses out to the left. Feel your body gently leaning over to the right. Press through your feet to ground yourself in the pose, particularly through your left foot,

5 ARDHA CHANDRASANA II YOGA MUDRA
Half-Moon II Seal of Yoga

Assume (4), with your back toes tucked in. Extend your arms behind your back, fingers interlaced. Keep your palms open as your arms lift up, away from your back.

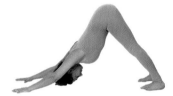

6 ARDHA DEVIJAI UTKATASANA
Half-Victory Goddess Squat

Bend your right knee, foot turned out. Extend your left leg. Your left foot faces forward. Bend both arms at right angles, palms facing inward, fingers spread. Bring your right arm out to the side, your left arm slightly in front.

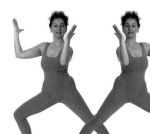

7 ARDHA MANDALASANA I
Half-Circle I

Ground your right shin and hand away from your buttock. Extend your left leg back, away from your right knee. Sweep your left arm up, to the right, lifting up your buttocks. Press your pointed left toes away from your left hip, your head away from your shoulders. Look up beyond your fingers.

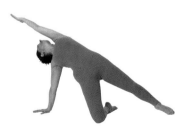

leg and hip. Allow your whole torso and both sides of your ribs to lift up and away from your pelvis, lengthening your chest. Engage your knees and legs.

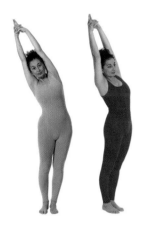

4 ARDHA CHANDRASANA II
Half-Moon II

With your right foot under your knee and your right calf at a right angle to your thigh, bring your left knee down, leg extended. Stretch back your left thigh as you press your left shin down into the ground. Keep your back leg pressed down, foot flat, and allow your hips to face forward. Lunge forward over your right leg. Feel your chest rise as you extend your arms outward into a V-shape, slightly softening the elbows to allow your shoulders to lower away from your ears (a). Lift your

head and chin and look up. Alternatively, extend your arms up vertically with palms together in *Namaskara* (Salutation) (b), as your head and chin also look up and your back arches.

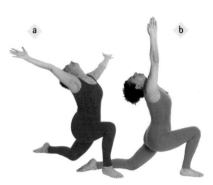

8 ARDHA MANDALASANA II
Half-Circle II

From (7), reach out your left arm to grasp your right waist. Lift your left leg up. Extend it out at a right angle with your left hip. Look ahead.

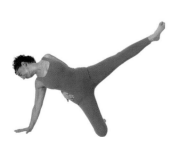

9 ARDHA MATSYENDRASANA I
Half-Spinal Twist I

Bend your right leg under you. Place your right foot along the outside of your left buttock. Cross your left leg to the outside of your right knee. Place your left foot along the outside of your right knee. Press your left palm to the ground, behind your back. Extend your right arm upward.

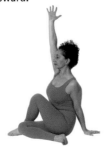

10 ARDHA MATSYENDRASANA II
Half-Spinal Twist II

From (9), hug your thigh on the outside of your left leg with your right arm. Together with your left hand, pressed into the ground, and your right arm, wedged against your left leg, leverage is created for your torso, abdomen, neck and head to rotate to the left. Keep your chin aligned with your left shoulder, both buttocks grounded.

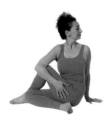

11 ARDHA NATARAJASANA II
Half-Dancer II
Balancing on your left leg, extend your left arm alongside your head. Bend your right arm and leg, elbow and knee touching each other. Rotate your right inner thigh and calf upward.

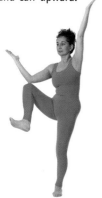

12 ARDHA PARSVOTTANASANA
Half-Pyramid
Bend your left leg, knee on the ground, left toes tucked in. Extend your right leg, foot flexed, fingers or palms touching the ground, either side of your right leg. Move your hips back, keeping them raised, as your chest comes to lie on your thighs.

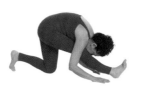

13 ARDHA SWASTIKASANA
Half-Cross
Bend your right leg, your foot at a right angle with your knee. Bend your left leg on the ground, aligned under your hip. Keep your chest vertical, arms out to the sides at shoulder level.

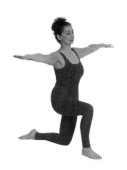

17 ASHWA SANCHALASANA II
Rider's II High Lunge
Bend your right leg with your knee and ankle forming right angles. Extend your left leg out behind you, toes tucked, keeping it straight and off the ground, while your left knee presses upward to create resistance. Press your hips down together to stretch your groin area. Keep your hands flat on the ground, both sides of your right foot.

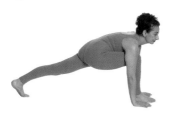

18 BHUJANGASANA
Cobra
Lie face down on the floor. Bend your elbows close by your sides, hands pressed on the ground, elbows bent under your shoulders. Using your back muscles initially, begin to lift up your torso, assisted by the push of your hands pressing into the ground. Lift up your head. Look up. Bring legs and heels together (advanced pose).

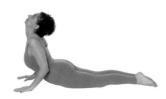

19 CHANDRA KONASANA
Moon Side Angle
Bend your right leg, calf and thigh, forming right angles. Bend your left leg behind you, at a right angle, foot flat. Extend your arms out at shoulder level. Tilt down to the right, fingertips touching the ground. Look beyond your left fingers.

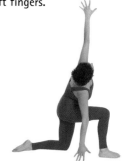

14 *ARDHA USHTRASANA CHANDRASANA*
Half-Camel Moon
Your right foot is on the ground at a right angle with your knee. Bend your left leg, knee under hip, left toes tucked in. Extend your right arm up and touch your left heel with your left hand.

15 *ARDHA VIRABHADRASANA II*
Half-Warrior II
As this pose is used dynamically in moving from side-to-side, your legs need to be spread with both feet turned out. Extend your arms out at shoulder level, bending your right knee as your torso moves toward the right and your head turns.

16 *ASHWA SANCHALASANA I*
Rider's I Lunge
Bend your right leg with your calf and thigh forming right angles. Extend your left leg out behind you, toes tucked in. Lunge your body forward over your right leg, fingertips touching the ground. Lift up your head as you stretch your groin area.

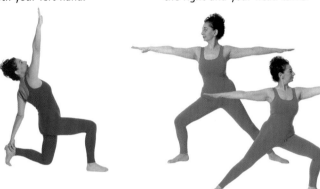

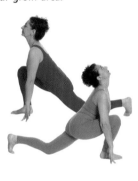

20 *DEVIJAI UTKATASANA*
Victory Goddess Squat
Spread your legs wide apart, bend your knees, your calves and thighs at right angles. Point your feet and toes outward. Bend your forearms and upper arms at right angles, palms half-facing outward, fingers spread. Activate your arms by pressing downward through your elbows. Energize your fingers by pressing them upward. Lower your shoulders down, away from your ears. Tuck your tailbone under, press your abdomen to your spine, as your body lowers to a comfortable squat. Look ahead, your tongue relaxed inside your mouth (a).

Alternatively you can look up to the space between your eyebrows in *Shambhavi Mudra* (Eyebrow Seal) to stimulate the energy center there. Extend your tongue from its roots down the length of your chin as far as you can (b).

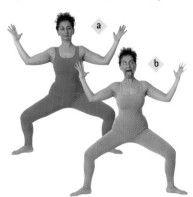

21 *DHANURASANA*
Bow
Bend your knees. Clasp your ankles with your hands. Keeping your arms straight, lift your head, torso and thighs off the ground as your feet press into your hands. Toes point upward, joining your big toes.

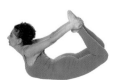

22 DHARMIKASANA
Hare/Extended Child
Sit on your heels and lay your torso flat over your thighs, resting your forehead on the ground. Extend your arms out in front, beyond your head, palms down. Bend your elbows slightly when using this pose for relaxation.

23 *EKAHASTAPADA MAJARIASANA*
One Hand-to-Foot Table Balance
From (43), bring your knees directly under your hips, wrists under your shoulders. Lift your right leg and extend it back as your right arm lifts and extends forward. Spread your fingers and toes. Balance your body and press deeply into your left shin muscles and left hand for support. Look ahead.

24 *EKAPADA CHANDRA NATARAJASANA I*
One-Foot Moon Dancer I
Bend your right leg forward, calf and thigh at right angles. Keep your left leg behind you, knee under hip, foot flat. Bring your body weight over your right leg. Reach your left hand back, clasping the top of your left foot, drawing it in toward your buttocks. Your right arm extends upward, fingers in *Gyan Mudra* (**Seal of Knowledge**).

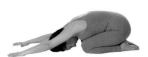

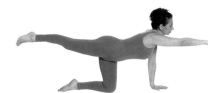

28 *EKAPADA DANDA MAJARIASANA*
One-Foot Table Press-Up
Keeping your chin, sternum and palms grounded, bend your elbows in toward the sides of your body. Extend your left leg upward, toes pointed, as your right knee, shin and the top of your foot remain grounded.

29 *EKAPADA JANU MAJARIASANA*
One-Foot Table Balance
Press your palms into the ground, fingers spread, balancing on your right knee and hands. Lift and extend your left leg. Lift your right foot to touch your left knee. Move your torso slightly forward, keeping elbows either bent or straight.

30 *GHARBHASANA*
Child
Fold your chest and abdomen over bent knees, feet flat. Touch your forehead to the ground in front of you, rest your arms alongside your body with your hands near your feet, palms facing upward. Your buttocks rest on your heels.

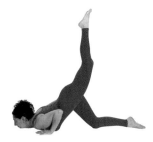

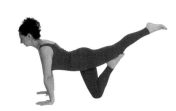

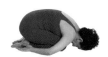

25 EKAPADA CHANDRA NATARAJASANA II
One-Foot Moon Dancer II
From (24), lunge your body forward, resting your chest on your right thigh as your right arm comes down to shoulder level in front of you.

26 EKAPADA CHANDRA NATARAJASANA III
One-Foot Moon Dancer III
From (25), reach both your hands out to clasp your left foot, fingers interlaced. Lift your head and open your throat and heart. Look upward as your foot presses into your hands and your back arches.

27 EKAPADA CHANDRA NATARAJASANA IV
One-Foot Moon Dancer IV
From (26), move your body weight forward. Bring your chest to the inside of your right thigh as your hands bring your left heel toward your left buttock. Balance on the top of your knee rather than mid-knee.

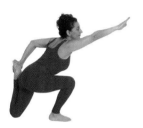

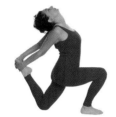

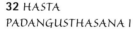

31 HALASANA
Plough
From a supine position, extend your legs up, over your body, beyond your head. Extend your arms behind your back, fingers interlaced, toes tucked in, legs straight.

32 HASTA PADANGUSTHASANA I
Hand-to-Foot Big Toe I
Balance your body on your left leg, left hand on your hip. Bend your right knee toward your chest with your index finger and thumb hooked around your big toe. Keep your chest vertical, chin parallel.

33 HASTA PADANGUSTHASANA II
Hand-to-Foot Big Toe II
Place your left hand on your left hip. Hook your right index finger and thumb around your right big toe, extending your right leg vertically in front of you. Keeping your right leg straight, chin parallel to the ground, tuck your tailbone in as you lengthen your torso upward.

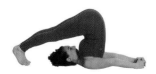

34 *HASTA UTTANASANA*
Raised Arms
Stand in (90). Extend your arms up and back, squeezing your buttocks to protect your lower back as your hips press forward. Open your arms out into a V-shape. Look up.

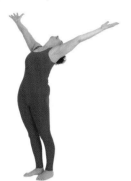

35 *HASTA UTTHAN VIRABHADRASANA II*
Warrior II Raised Arm
Bend your right leg, your knee at a right angle with your ankle. Extend your right arm up, alongside your face. Keep your left leg straight, left foot turned out. Line up both heels. Bring your left arm down by your side. Stretch your body up, slightly to the left. Look ahead.

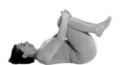
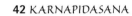

36 *JANU JHULANASANA*
Sacral-Rocking
Lying on your back, hold your knees in toward your chest, fingers interlaced around your knees. Rock your body gently from side-to-side, feeling your sacrum and lumbar spine being massaged.

40 *KAKASANA*
Crow
Keep your palms flat, fingers spread, elbows bent, your shins resting on the backs of your upper arms, close to your armpits, feet off the ground, soles together. Look along the ground. Straighten your arms.

41 *KAPOTASANA*
Pigeon
Bend your right leg, your foot and heel in toward your right groin. Extend your left leg behind your body, foot flat. Place your hands on the ground for balance. Face forward and open your heart and chest. Lift up your chin as your hands press into the ground and your back arches.

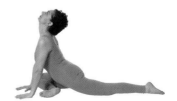

42 *KARNAPIDASANA*
Ear Pressure
From (31), bring your knees down beside your ears. Press into them. Bring your knees farther down to touch the ground by the sides of your shoulders. Keep your forearms on the backs of your thighs. Thread your hands under your head and cup them over your ears. Press your elbows toward the ground.

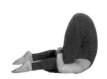

37 JANU MANDALASANA
Knee-Circling

Lie on your back with your hands on top of your knees. Guide both knees, initially clockwise, then anticlockwise, in a circling motion.

38 JANU SIRSHASANA I
Head-to-Knee I

Bend your right leg, the sole of your right foot pressing into your left inner thigh, left leg extended, foot flexed. Keep your torso vertical. Raise your arms up by your temples.

39 JANU SIRSHASANA II
Head-to-Knee II

Keeping your legs as in (38), rest your abdomen and torso on your left thigh. Bend your left leg and bring your knee to your forehead. Place your hands either side of your left foot (a) or clasp your left foot, fingers interlaced (b). Press your right knee into the ground as your left heel presses away.

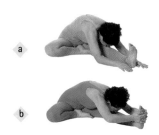

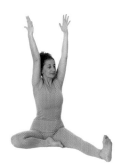

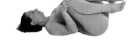

43 MAJARIASANA
Table

Come down on all fours, your knees hip-width apart. Place them under your hips, hands parallel, shoulder-width apart, palms flat, fingers spread, wrists under your shoulders. Press the crown of your head away from your tailbone (a). For Cat Tilt, press your hands into the ground as you round your back, lowering your head down, chin to throat (b).

44 MAJARIASANA JANU SIRSHASANA
Table Head-to-Knee

From (43), ground your left leg and your left hand. Extend your right leg out to the side in line with your right hip. Balance your left palm and leg by grounding them. Look at your right big toe. Hook it with the first two fingers of your right hand. Move your head toward your right knee.

45 MANIPURASANA
Abdominal

Position both legs perpendicular to your torso, feet flexed. Keep your arms parallel to the ground, palms facing down. Lift your chest and arms toward your thighs.

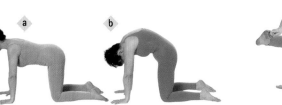

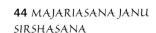

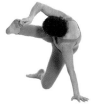

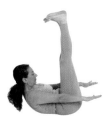

46 *MATSYASANA*
Fish
Place your arms underneath your buttocks, palms flat, legs extended, feet pointed. Rest the top of your head on the ground, arching your back and bringing the curve up behind your heart as your chest expands upward. Press down your palms, forearms and buttocks to maintain the upward movement of your chest.

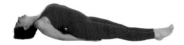

47 *NAMASKARA CHANDRASANA*
Salutation to the Moon
Bend your right leg with your calf and thigh forming right angles. Bend your left leg at a right angle, foot flat. Keep your torso vertical, arms out in front of your body at shoulder level, palms together, fingers pressing forward.

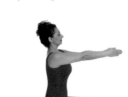

48 *NAMASKARA PARIVRTTA PARSVAKONASANA I*
Revolved Salutation Side Angle I
Bend your right leg, your calf and thigh forming right angles. Bend your left leg at a right angle. Rotate your torso to the right, lay your chest against the inside of your right thigh, elbows bent, palms in *Namaskara* (Salutation) in front of your heart. Look over your right shoulder.

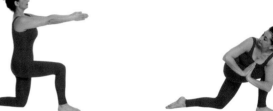

51 *NATARAJASANA II*
Dancer II
Bend your left leg, turn your foot out. Raise your right leg and bend your knee, foot flexed. Bend your right elbow with the back of your hand in front of your forehead. Bend your left elbow, palm facing outward and downward, toward your right foot.

52 *PADA HASTASANA*
Standing Hand-to-Foot Forward Fold
Fold your body in half, hinging from your hips. Your hands touch the ground, either side of your feet. Keep palms flat, fingers spread, aligned with your toes, and press them into the ground. Bring your torso and thighs together, bending your knees if necessary, leaving no gap between them.

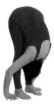
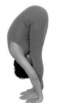

53 *PANCHANGASANA*
Five-Pointed Star
Spread your legs, feet pointing outward. Extend your arms out into a V-shape. Turn arms and palms in, palms facing back. Your body "looks" like a cross or a star with the intersection at the heart.

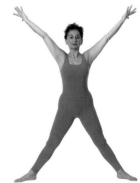

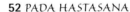

49 *NAMASKARA PARIVRTTA PARSVAKONASANA II*
Revolved Salutation Side Angle II
Bend your right leg, your calf and thigh forming right angles. Extend your left leg behind you, foot flat and turned in, heels aligned. Rotate your trunk until your left armpit is wedged against the outside of your right knee. Bend your elbows with palms in *Namaskara* (Salutation) in front of your heart. Look over your right shoulder.

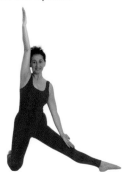

50 *NATARAJASANA I*
Dancer I
Balancing on your left leg, ground your left foot. Extend your right leg upward, behind you, away from your buttock, with your right hand holding the outside of your right foot. Spread your toes. Extend your left arm in front, above shoulder level, your thumb and index finger joined together in *Gyan Mudra* (Seal of Knowledge). Ensure that both your hips are squared to the front before moving your body forward. Roll your right hip forward and your left hip backward. With your hips rotating to the front, press your right foot into your right hand.

With your right hand gently resisting your right foot, move your body toward the horizontal. Look up at your fingertips (a) or look down (b).

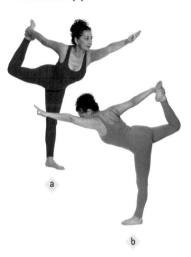

54 *PARIGHASANA I*
Gate I
From a kneeling position, extend your left leg out to the side, your sole on the ground, foot pointed, left heel aligned with your right knee. Rest your left arm on your left leg, palm facing up. Extend your right arm upward.

55 *PARIGHASANA II*
Gate II
From (54), lean your trunk over toward the left with your palms eventually moving toward each other. Move your upper arms and shoulders back as your trunk rotates forward and upward.

56 *PARIGHASANA III*
Gate III
From a kneeling position, extend your left leg out to the side, sole flat, foot pointed. Lean your torso slowly to the right as your right palm touches the ground. Extend your left arm alongside your ear. Lean your body to the right. Look up.

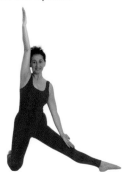

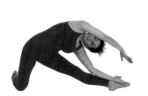

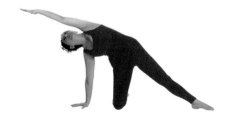

57 PARIVRTTA ARDHA CHANDRASANA
Revolved Half-Moon

Bend your right knee, calf and thigh at a right angle. Bend your left leg, knee down, foot flat. Wedge your left arm against the outside of your right knee. Rotate your torso to the right. Extend your right arm behind you at shoulder level. Look beyond your right fingers.

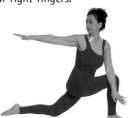

58 PARIVRTTA ARDHA USHTRASANA CHANDRASANA
Revolved Half-Camel Moon

Bend your right knee, calf and thigh at a right angle. Bend your left leg, knee down, toes tucked in. Reach your right hand back and touch your left heel. Extend your left arm up as your back arches and your heart opens. Look up beyond your left hand.

59 PARIVRTTA CHANDRA KONASANA
Revolved Moon Side Angle

Bend your right knee, your calf and thigh at a right angle. Bend your left leg, knee down, foot flat. Extend your arms out at shoulder level as your torso rotates to the right. Look beyond your right hand.

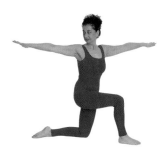

63 PARSVOTTANASANA II
Pyramid II

As in (62), only place your hands behind your back in *Namaskara* (Salutation). Keep your heart open, shoulders back, your elbows lifted, your chin towards or on your shin.

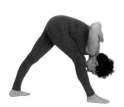

64 PARSVOTTANASANA YOGA MUDRA I
Pyramid Seal of Yoga I

Spread your legs, turn your torso and feet to the left. Line up your torso over your left leg. Interlace your hands behind your back and lift them up off your back as your trunk comes to horizontal.

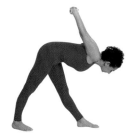

65 PARSVOTTANASANA YOGA MUDRA II
Pyramid Seal of Yoga II

As in (64), only lay your trunk toward or on your left leg with your arms extended up off your back.

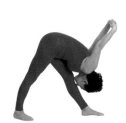

60 *PARIVRTTA UTTHITA TRIKONASANA*
Revolved Extended Triangle
Spread your legs, right foot out at a right angle, left foot in. Align both heels. Engage kneecaps and thighs. Rest your left fingertips or palm on the ground on the outside of your right foot. Extend your right arm up, align your shoulders. Press your left arm against your right leg to rotate your torso to the right.

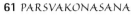

61 *PARSVAKONASANA*
Lateral Angle
Bend your right knee, calf and thigh at a right angle. Extend your left leg, foot turned in, heels aligned. Rest your right palm on the outside of your right foot. Extend your left arm by your face, palm down. Look beyond your left fingers. Rotate your torso, aligning it with your hips and legs.

62 *PARSVOTTANASANA I*
Pyramid I
Spread your legs, turn your torso and feet to the right. Rotate your torso over your right leg and lay it flat over your right thigh, palms or fingertips touching the ground, either side of your foot. Keep both legs straight and engage your knees and thighs.

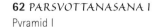

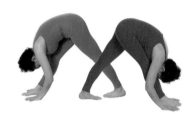

66 *PASCHIMOTTANASANA*
Seated Forward Fold
From a sitting position, extend your legs in front of your body, feet flexed. Hook your big toes with your index and second fingers, or rest your hands on your legs, shins or ankles. Lay your torso on your thighs, hinging forward from your hips, with your chin toward your shins.

67 *PAVANMUKTASANA I*
Wind-Relieving I
Bend your right knee against your abdomen with both hands clasped around the outside of your knee. Draw it toward your chest. Extend your left leg away from you with the back of your leg pressing down to the ground. Flex both feet.

68 *PAVANMUKTASANA II*
Wind-Relieving II
As in (67), only bring your head up toward your knee.

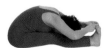

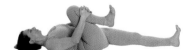

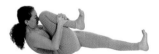

69 *POORNA HRIDAYASANA*
Full Heart
Bend your right leg, your foot at a right angle to your knee. Bend your left leg, foot flat, keeping your knee on the ground, aligned under your hip. Hold your arms out at shoulder level, palms up, and move back slightly as your heart opens.

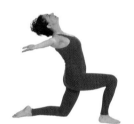

70 *PRANAMASANA*
Prayer
Stand with feet hip-width apart and bring your pelvis into a neutral position (almost Cat Tilt), feet parallel, palms together in front of your heart in *Namaskara* (Salutation). Look ahead.

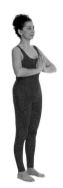
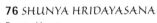

71 *PRASARITA PADOTTANASANA*
Spread-Leg Forward Fold
Spread both legs and engage your kneecaps and thighs, keeping your feet parallel. Extend your trunk forward with your palms on the ground, fingers spread, elbows at right angles with your wrists. Press your hands into the ground, drawing your torso through your legs. Touch the crown of your head to the ground.

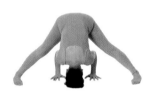

75 *SETHU BANDHASANA*
Bridge
Keep your feet parallel and hip-width apart. With your pelvis in Cat Tilt, lift upward, arching your back, arms extended on the ground beyond your head, chin tucked in toward your throat.

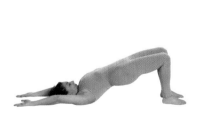

76 *SHUNYA HRIDAYASANA*
Empty Heart
Bend your right leg, your foot at a right angle with your knee. Bend your left leg, keeping your knee on the ground, aligned under your hip. Round your back, bringing your arms forward, palms pressed together, fingers pressing away, your chin tucked in toward your throat.

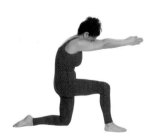

77 *SPHINXASANA*
Sphinx
Keeping your legs hip-width apart, rest your forearms on the ground, elbows under each shoulder, palms down, fingers spread. Your elbows are at right angles to your shoulders. Keep your chin parallel to the ground and open your heart, your abdomen tucked in, pelvis in Cat Tilt.

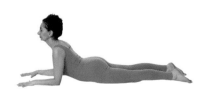

72 *PRASARITA PADOTTANASANA YOGA MUDRA*
Spread-Leg Forward Fold
Seal of Yoga
As (71), but bring your hands behind your back, fingers interlaced. Raise your arms up off your back.

73 *SALAMBA KAKASANA*
Inverted Crow
Place the crown of your head on the ground. Spread your hands and fingers. Your head and hands form an equilateral triangle with your head as the peak. Bend your elbows at right angles with your wrists. Rest your knees on the backs of your upper arms, feet off the ground. Balance. Bring the soles of your feet together.

74 *SAVASANA*
Corpse
Lie flat on your back, legs and inner thighs apart, arms out to the sides, away from your body, palms up. Elongate your neck, tuck your chin in toward your throat, close your eyes, relax your facial muscles. Align head and spine.

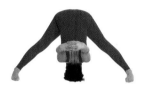

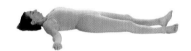

78 *STHITHI PAVANMUKTASANA I*
Standing Wind-Relieving I
Keeping your body grounded by engaging your supporting leg, place your left hand on your left hip for balance. Pull up on your left kneecap and thigh, engaging your pelvic floor and firming up your lower abdomen. Elongate your back, press the crown of your head upward and keep your neck long for a full spinal stretch. Bend your right leg as you gently bring your right knee in toward your chest, your pelvis in Cat Tilt.

Clasp either one hand (a) or both hands (b) around the outside of your right knee, your fingers interlaced, foot flexed, your toes spread. Look ahead.

79 *STHITHI PAVANMUKTASANA II*
Standing Wind-Relieving II
As (78), but with your left hand on your left hip. Turn your right leg out to the right, your knee held up by your right hand.

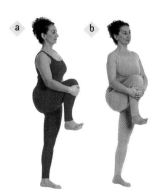

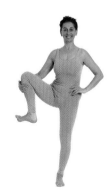

80 SUKHASANA
Easy
Cross your legs, keeping your back vertical, your hands on your knees or in your lap. Relax your arms. Press the crown of your head upward. Align your neck, head and spine. Look ahead.

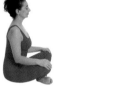

81 SUPTA ARDHA PADMASANA
Supine Half-Lotus
Bend your left leg, keeping the sole of your foot flat on the ground. Bend your right leg, crossing it over your left thigh. Turn the sole of your foot upward. Press your right knee down as far as you can. Your left hand holds the toes of your right foot and your right hand gently eases your right knee downward.

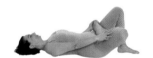

82 SUPTA EKAPADASANA
Supine Single-Leg Reclining Lunge
Bend your left leg, keeping the sole of your foot flat on the ground. Lift and bend your right leg, your calf forming a right angle with your right thigh. Clasp your hands around the flexed sole of your right foot. With your hands, gently ease your knee down toward the ground beside your chest. Keeping your shoulders down, open your heart and ground your sacrum. Align your neck and spine.

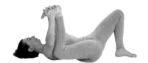

86 SUPTA UTTANPADASANA/ MANDALASANA
Supine Single-Leg Raising/Circling
With your arms out at shoulder level, palms down on the ground, raise your right leg upward. With your foot pointed, begin circling your leg around in one direction, then the other, ensuring the action comes from your hip, keeping your left leg extended along the ground.

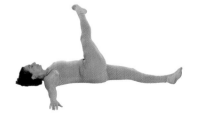

87 SUPTA VRKSHASANA
Supine Tree
Extend your left leg away from you, foot flexed. Bend your right leg and place the sole of your foot along the inside of your left thigh. Bring your pelvis into Cat Tilt to smooth out your lower back arch and move your right knee toward the ground. Extend your arms up beyond your head, hands in *Namaskara* (Salutation).

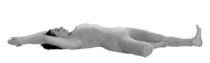

88 SUTRA HASTA MAJARIASANA I
Threading-the-Needle I
From (43), ground your left hand, palm down, fingers spread, as your right arm threads through the gap between your left knee and hand. Bring your right shoulder and the back of your head down to the ground. Look up.

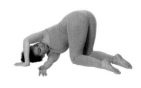

83 *SUPTA KAPOTASANA*
Supine Pigeon
Bend your right leg under your chest. Drawing your heel in toward your right groin, extend your left leg out behind your body, toes out. Lay your torso over your right thigh, extending your arms out in front, palms down, forehead to the ground.

84 *SUPTA MATSYENDRASANA*
Supine Knee-Down Twist
Rotate your body to the left so your shoulder, hip, knee and ankle are aligned. Extend your left leg, foot pointed. Bend your right leg. Your right foot rests on your left knee; your left hand rests on the outside of your right knee. Ease your knee down to the ground. Ground your right shoulder. Turn your head to the right.

85 *SUPTA PADANGUSTHASANA*
Supine Hand-to-Foot
Bend your left leg, keeping the sole of your foot flat on the ground. Extend your right leg upward. Hook your right index and second finger around the big toe of your right foot. Extend your left arm, resting your left hand on your left thigh.

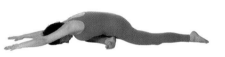
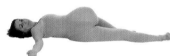
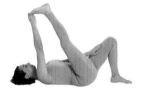

89 *SUTRA HASTA MAJARIASANA II*
Threading-the-Needle II
From (88), extend your left leg out behind your body, your foot pointed and grounded. Lift your left arm and extend it up and back, keeping it on the ground, opening your heart and chest. Keep your neck relaxed and your shoulders grounded.

90 *TADASANA I*
Mountain I
Keep your body upright, feet parallel and hip-width apart, engage kneecaps and thighs to distribute your weight evenly through your legs and feet. Bring your arms down by your sides, away from your body, palms facing in, fingers spread. Press the crown of your head upward, release your shoulders, tuck your tailbone in, your pelvis in Cat Tilt. Look ahead.

91 *TADASANA II*
Mountain II
As (90), and extend your arms up alongside your ears. With fingers pointing upward, spread palms and fingers, drop your shoulders down, away from your ears. Extend your arms upward as your shoulders move down.

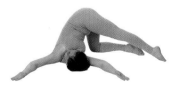
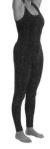

92 *TADASANA III*
Mountain III
As (90), and interlace your hands above your head, turning your palms out.

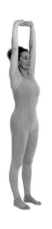

93 *TALASANA I*
Mountain I Variation
Come up on tiptoes. Extend your right arm upward. Circle it behind you. Return it to the side as your heels come down to the ground.

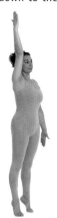

94 *TALASANA II*
Mountain II Variation
As (93), and extend both your arms upward.

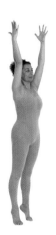

98 *URDHVA EKAPADAJANU MAJARIASANA*
Upward One-Foot Hip Press
Begin in (43), and bend your right knee, calf and thigh at a right angle, foot flexed. Press the sole of your foot upward. Feel the action coming from your hip.

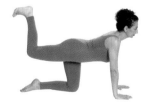

99 *URDHVA EKAPADA MAJARIASANA I*
Upward One-Foot Leg Table I
From (98), place both wrists beneath your shoulders, left knee beneath your hip, right leg out to the side, foot flexed, parallel to the ground, aligned with your right hip. Look at your right big toe. Swing your right leg back, foot pointed, hips aligned, as you look ahead. Swing your leg back to the side. Look at your big toe.

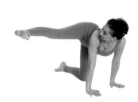

100 *URDHVA EKAPADA MAJARIASANA II*
Upward One-Foot Leg Table II
Begin as (98). Extend your right leg out to the side. Look at your right big toe. Press into your left shin and palm. Reach your right big toe with your right hand. Hook it with your right index and second fingers. Keep your leg parallel to the ground (a) or lift it up higher (b) for a fuller stretch.

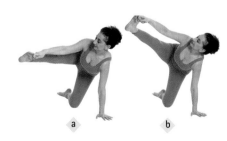

95 *TALASANA III*
Mountain III Variation
Come up on tiptoes, arms out to the sides. Bring palms together in *Namaskara* (Salutation) above your head. Circle them back behind you.

96 *TALASANA IV*
Mountain IV Variation
Cross your wrists in front of your pelvis. Come up on tiptoes. Reach your arms out and up to vertical. Separate and circle your arms back behind you as they reach the sides of your body.

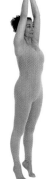

97 *UBBAYA PADANGUSTHASANA*
Raised Big Toes
Balancing on your tailbone, extend your legs upward, engaging your kneecaps and thighs, arms straight, and extend forward toward your feet. Hook the index and second finger of each hand around the big toe of each of your feet. Keep your back straight, pelvis in Dog Tilt. Look at your big toes, your body in a V-shape.

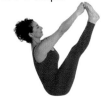

101 *URDHVA EKAPADAJANU CHAKRA MAJARIASANA*
Upward One-Foot Hip Rotation
Begin as (98), only bend your right leg at the knee, foot flexed, your calf and thigh at right angles. Rotate your knee in one direction, then the other. Feel the action coming from your hip.

102 *URDHVA HANUMANASANA*
Upward-Standing Splits
Take this pose in stages. Balance on your right leg, toes spread, palms flat, fingers spread, alongside your foot (advanced pose). Create a triangle with your foot and hands. Keep your hips level to avoid twisting out to the side. Lay your torso on your right thigh, leaving no gap between your chest and thighs, chin toward your shin. Extend your left leg as high up as you can, almost to vertical (a). Engage thighs and kneecaps. If this is too challenging, bend your right leg to a slight angle, lifting your left leg

to just above horizontal (b). For a more basic stretch, lift your left leg to just below horizontal, knee slightly bent (c).

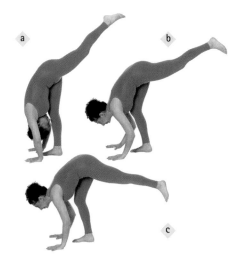

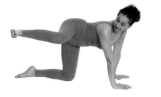

103 URDHVA HANUMANASANA YOGA MUDRA
Upward-Standing Splits Seal of Yoga
As (102), but with your arms behind your back, fingers interlaced. Lift them off your back. Merge your chest and thighs, chin toward your shin.

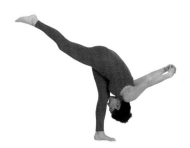

104 URDHVA MUKHA SVANASANA
Upward-Facing Dog
Support and balance your body on your hands and toes. Keep your wrists beneath your shoulders, palms flat, fingers spread. Press into the ground, feet hip-width apart, toes tucked in. Extend your legs off the ground, engaging kneecaps and thighs. Roll back your shoulders, lift up your head and chin. Look up.

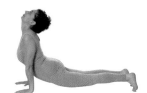

105 URDHVA VAJRASANA
Upward Thunderbolt
Sit on your heels. Lift your head and arms upward. Open your heart. Look up. Arch your back slightly and open your arms out into a V-shape.

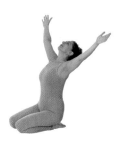

109 UTTHAN PRISTHASANA I
Lizard I
Assume a prone position, folding your arms under your chest with each of your hands holding onto an elbow. Open your chest and heart. Look up. Keep your legs hip-width apart, feet extended, and your elbows stable as you press into them.

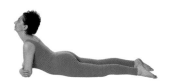

110 UTTAN PRISTHASANA II
Lizard II
From (109), press your elbows, forearms and knees into the ground as you lift up your buttocks. Move back to align them above your knees. Bring your chest toward the ground, keeping your chin or forehead grounded.

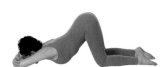

111 UTTHITA EKAPADA ANGUSTHASANA
Extended One-Leg Tiptoe
Bend your left knee, foot flat on the ground. Extend your right leg out in front, parallel to the ground, knees together. Clasp both hands around the outside of your right foot. To balance, initially hold the outside of your right foot with your right hand while your left hand touches the ground at the side.

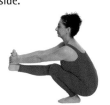

106 *USHTRASANA*
Camel
From a kneeling position, keeping your thighs parallel and hip-width apart, bring your pelvis into Cat Tilt, with toes out or toes tucked in (easier pose). Both your hands reach back to rest on your heels or feet. Open your heart, pressing your pelvis and hips forward. Your head can be in a forward position, or lifted up and back. Look up or behind you.

107 *UTKATASANA I*
Standing Squat I
Keeping your torso vertical, feet flat, hold your arms out horizontally in front of your body at shoulder level. Bend your knees as you lower down to a squat as if to sit down on a chair.

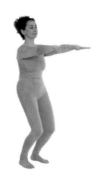

108 *UTKATASANA II*
Standing Squat II
As (107), only lift your heels off the ground, coming up on tiptoes for balance. The squat is exactly the same, only on tiptoes.

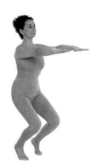

112 *UTTHITA EKAPADASANA*
Raised One-Foot I
Balancing on your left leg, extend your right leg out in front, foot pointed. Extend your arms up alongside your ears.

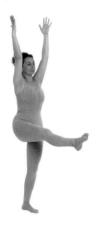

113 *UTTHITA EKAPADASANA II*
Raised One-Foot II
Balancing on your left leg, keep your trunk horizontal. Extend your right leg out behind you, foot flexed, hips aligned to avoid any tipping or lifting up. Extend your arms out to horizontal at shoulder level. Look down.

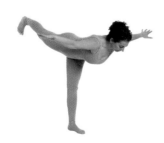

114 *UTTHITA EKAPADA MAJARIASANA*
Extended One-Foot Table
From (43), place your wrists beneath your shoulders, palms flat, fingers spread. Look ahead. Lift up your right leg and extend it behind you, foot pointed. Balance.

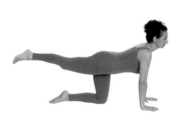

115 *UTTHITA TRIKONASANA*
Extended Triangle

Spread your legs. Turn your right foot out at a right angle, your left foot in. Align your heels. Engage both your kneecaps and thighs. Press the back of your left heel away from you, with toes slightly turned in. Reach over to the right. Extend your torso vertically and your arms horizontally. Extend both arms away from each other. Keeping your spine straight, tilt your arms downward. Reach your right palm or fingers toward your right ankle, shin or

thigh on the inside of your right foot. Extend your left arm up vertically, aligning it with your right shoulder. Spread your fingers. Look up at your left hand. Keep your trunk horizontal, your legs forming an equilateral triangle beneath it.

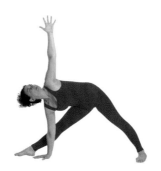

11 *VAJRASANA*
Thunderbolt

Sit on your heels, knees together, your hands resting on your thighs, palms down (a), or in *Namaskara* (Salutation) (b). Keep your torso vertical, your pelvis in soft Cat Tilt. Avoid arching your spine. Keep your chin parallel to the ground. Look ahead.

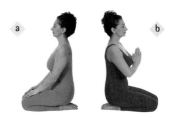

119 *VRKSHASANA*
Tree

Look ahead. Center your weight evenly over both legs. Balance on your left leg, engaging kneecap and thigh, toes spread, sole pressing into the ground. Place your right foot inside your left inner thigh as high up as you can, pelvis in Cat Tilt, palms in *Namaskara* (Salutation), either in front of your heart, with elbows bent (a), on the crown of your head, with elbows bent outward (b), or in full pose, with arms extended above your head (c). If you are new to this pose, the lowest your right foot can be is with your right big toe placed on

the ground, your foot flat along your heel and ankle, your right knee pointing outward. Gradually move your foot up your leg and into your left inner thigh.

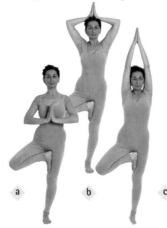

120 *YOGA MUDRA I*
Seal of Yoga I

Sit in (116), your arms behind your back. Interlace your fingers, opening your chest and heart. Lift up your chin.

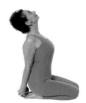

117 *VIRABHADRASANA I*
Warrior I
Spread your legs, turning your right foot at a right angle. Bend your knee, calf and thigh at right angles. Turn your left foot in, extend your leg, engaging your kneecap and thigh. Rotate your torso to face over your right leg, keeping both hips forward. Extend your arms upward, palms together. Look up.

118 *VIRABHADRASANA II*
Warrior II
Spread your legs and align your heels, your calf and thigh at right angles. Turn your left foot in, your heel slightly pressing away, your toes turned in. Press into the outer edge of your left foot. Extend your left leg and engage your kneecap and thigh. Extend your arms sideways to shoulder level, fingers spread. Keep your torso stationary and facing forward. Look beyond your right fingers.

Lower your pelvis downward as your fingers and arms press away from each other and your right knee bends deeper. Allow your left hip to comfortably roll back as you stretch your groin area.

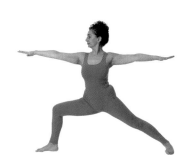

121 *YOGA MUDRA II*
Seal of Yoga II
From (120), lean your trunk forward over your thighs with your buttocks on your heels. Extend your arms off your back in an upward motion. Place your forehead on the ground, keeping your shoulders back and away from your ears.

122 *YOGA MUDRA III*
Seal of Yoga III
From (121), lift your buttocks off your heels, moving upward. Roll onto the top of your head.

123 *YOGA MUDRA IV*
Seal of Yoga IV
From (122), extend your right leg out behind you, pressing deeply into your left shin and foot as well as your right foot. Feel the pressure going down through the crown of your head.

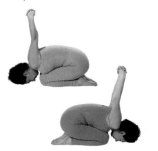

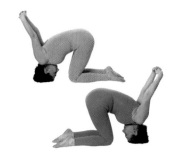

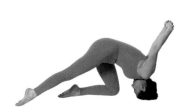

index

Yoga Poses

acknowledgments

To my students for being open to the newness of yogaflows and for contributing life to form through their feedback and support.

To Amy Carroll and Denise Brown for your belief in yogaflows and all staff at Carroll and Brown: especially, my editor, Anna Amari-Parker, for your encouragement, certainty and confidence; Evie Loizides-Graham, for your creativity; photographer Jules Selmes, for your professionalism and humor.

To all my teachers, from whom I have been blessed to receive guidance and support, and whose direct knowledge and experience have inspired me to move deeper within myself: especially, Sri Mata Amritanandamayi Ma, for your love; Sri HRL Poonjaji, for your wisdom and laughter; Swami Shri Kripalvanandji, Yogi Amrit Desai and Mickey Singer, for your unique distillation of the great teachings; Erich Schiffmann, Andrea Durant and Ruth Allen, for your authenticity and inspiration.

To my family and friends who have loved, encouraged and supported me: especially, Gilli Dawson, for knowing how to rejoice and for your advice on the text; Rita Mitra, for your strength and spirit; MJ Bindu Delekta, for your depth; Renée Found, for your feedback on the text, and my brother, Ram Chatlani. Special thanks to Judith Durgati Medhurst, for your constancy and untiring help in understanding and feeling the work.

Thank you to my parents, Renée and Rewa: their love, heritage and support have contributed greatly to who I am and made all of this possible by bringing me into this world. To the Spirit for manifesting yogaflows. I am humbled by the Grace I feel. May all of you be blessed by Love, our deepest and truest nature.

Love, Mohini

Carroll & Brown would like to thank:

Production manager
Karol Davies

Production controller
Nigel Reed

Computer management
Paul Stradling

Indexer
Madeline Weston

Unitards by **Marie Wright** at www.mariewright.net. All other clothes: author's own.

Resources
For further information on yogaflows, classes, retreats and Mohini's teaching schedule, visit *www.heartspaceyoga.com.*